Khaoula Rekik
Ranim Toumi
Mounir Ben Jemaa

Management of necrotizing otitis externa

Khaoula Rekik
Ranim Toumi
Mounir Ben Jemaa

Management of necrotizing otitis externa

News

ScienciaScripts

Cover image: www.ingimage.com

This book is a translation from the original published under ISBN 978-620-6-72308-0.

Publisher:
Sciencia Scripts
is a trademark of
Dodo Books Indian Ocean Ltd. and OmniScriptum S.R.L publishing group

120 High Road, East Finchley, London, N2 9ED, United Kingdom
Str. Armeneasca 28/1, office 1, Chisinau MD-2012, Republic of Moldova, Europe
Printed at: see last page
ISBN: 978-620-8-33580-9

CONTENTS

LIST OF ABBREVIATIONS

ADP	Adenopathy
Amox-Ac Clav	Amoxicillin-clavulanic acid
TMJ	Temporomandibular joint
C3G	3rd generation cephalosporins
CAE	External auditory canal
CRP:	C reactive protein
DID	Insulin-dependent diabetes
NIDDM	Non-insulin-dependent diabetes
FDG PET/CT	Fluorodeoxyglucose Positron Emission Tomography
Ga67	Gallium 67
Gado	Gadolinium
Hb	Hemoglobin
HbA1c	Glycated hemoglobin
HC	Blood culture
HTA	High blood pressure
IgA	Immunoglobulin A
IgG	Immunoglobulin G
IM	Intramuscular
MRI	Magnetic resonance imaging
IV	Intravenous
CBC	Blood count
OE	Otitis externa
OEN	Necrotizing external otitis
HBOT	hyperbaric oxygen therapy
OR	Odds Ratio
ENT	Otolaryngology
PFP	Peripheral facial palsy
pH	Hydrogen potential

RCAE	External auditory canal stricture
MRSA	Methicillin-resistant Staphylococcus aureus
AIDS	Acquired Immune Deficiency Syndrome
SPECT	Single-photon emission computed tomography
Tc99m	Technétium 99m
CT SCAN	Computed tomography
PET/CT	Positron emission tomography/computed tomography
HIV	Human Immunodeficiency Virus
VO	Oral route
VS	Sedimentation rate

INTRODUCTION

Infections of the external ear, commonly known as otitis externa (OE), are one of the most common disorders of the ear canal. Although most cases are benign, and usually resolve with well-managed local treatment within 15 days (1), there is a rare but serious form of the condition: necrotizing otitis externa (NEO). It was first described in 1959 by Meltzer and Kelemen (2). In 1968, J.R. Chandler identified and named this pathology "malignant otitis externa" (3). The term "malignant" is not linked to its neoplastic origin, but rather to its fatal outcome.

Characterized by rapid destruction of the tissues of the external auditory canal (EAC), OEN can progress to full-blown osteitis of the skull base, with potentially devastating forms extending to the deep soft tissues of the face and central nervous system (4).

Despite advances in medicine, necrotizing otitis externa continues to present a major challenge to the clinician in terms of early diagnosis, effective treatment, prognosis and prevention (5).

Its incidence has risen significantly in recent decades, arousing growing interest in the medical community.

OEN usually occurs in elderly diabetic subjects, especially men or immunocompromised subjects, but not exclusively (5).

The clinical picture often combines otalgia resistant to analgesics and local treatments, hypoacusis and ± purulent otorrhea. The germ most frequently found is *Pseudomonas aeruginosa* (6).

This entity jeopardizes the hearing health of individuals, leading to a rapid deterioration in patients' quality of life and imposing a considerable economic burden on healthcare systems. Hence the importance of a better understanding of its epidemiology, mechanisms and early diagnosis options for optimal management.

CHAPTER 1:
EPIDEMIOLOGICAL STUDY

1. FREQUENCY

Initially uncommon and rarely documented in the literature, OEN has seen an increase in incidence in recent years (Table XVIII).

Table I: Frequency of necrotizing otitis externa in the literature

Study	Number of cases	Study duration (years)	Location
Chen (7)	55	22 (1990-2011)	Taiwan
Hamzany (8)	60	19 (1990-2008)	Petah Tikva
Chintiri (9)	45	10 (1994-2003)	Tunisia
Cheng (10)	773	15 (2001-2015)	Taiwan
Guerrero-Espejo (11)	355	6 (2008-2013)	Spain
Arsovic (12)	30	10 (2008- 2018)	Serbia
Hatch (13)	786*	3 (2012-2015)	United States
Eweiss (14)	39	8 (2012-2020)	United Kingdom

*Patients hospitalized in 187 US hospitals.

2. ANNUAL BREAKDOWN

The incidence of OEN worldwide is not well documented and may vary according to region, populations studied and diagnostic criteria used. Chawdhary et al (15) showed a six-fold increase in the number of cases between 1999 (n = 67) and 2013 (n = 421), Bhasker et al (16) showed a statistically significant increase in the frequency of diagnosis of SDO during the study period (p = 0.0027) from 2004 to 2012 and Eweiss et al (14) showed an increase in the number of SDO cases from 9 cases (2012-2016) to 30 cases (2016-2020). All these studies were conducted in the UK. This growing trend can be explained by increased awareness of the disease, an ageing population and the rising prevalence of diabetes. A few studies have shown a stable incidence of SDO over the years (17).

To obtain precise estimates of the incidence of SDO worldwide, more extensive epidemiological studies would be required.

3. INCIDENCE BY AGE

The incidence of OEN is higher in subjects aged 65 or over (10) (18) (Table XIX).

However, this condition is not confined to the elderly; it can also be seen in young people, particularly those suffering from acquired immunodeficiency syndrome (AIDS).

Table II: Average age according to various series in the literature

Study	Year	Average age (years)	Extreme (years)
Sylvester (17)	2016	54,1	-
Hutson and Watson (19)	2019	72	40-89
Arsovic (12)	2020	71	52-88
Costa (20)	2023	69,5	61-76,7
In Tunisia			
Chnitir (9)	2005	67	50-84
Abed (21)	2016	66,5	48-86

4. DISTRIBUTION BY GENDER

Most studies have noted a male predominance (12) (22) (20) (Table XX).

This can be explained, on the one hand, by the fact that the hydrogen potential (pH) of earwax is less acidic in men than in women, which would reduce its antibacterial action in the ear, and, on the other hand, by poor compliance with diabetes treatment, which is more frequent in men than in women.

A predominance of women was noted in some studies:

- ❖ Yiğider et al (23) had a series of 26 patients including 17 women and 9 men.
- ❖ Sylvester et al (24) had a series of 8200 cases, 52.2% of which were women and 47.8% men.

Table III: Gender distribution of patients in the literature

Study	Number of cases	Men	Women	Sex ratio
Nenad et al (12)	30	27	3	9
Guevara et al (22)	22	17	5	3,4
Sideris et al (25)	36	27	9	3
Guerrero-Espejo et al (11)	355	250	105	2,4

5. GEOGRAPHICAL ORIGIN

To date, studies on the correlation between geographical origin and the incidence of OEN remain insufficient. Some studies have shown a higher incidence in rural areas (26). Other studies have shown a predominance in hot, humid regions (27).

CHAPTER 2:
CLINICAL STUDY

1. ASSOCIATED FACTORS

In the literature, several factors have been associated with OEN. It is important to note that the presence of one or more of these factors is inconsistent: Significant exposure to water (swimming or diving) or forced introduction into the EAC of water contaminated with *Pseudomonas aeruginosa*, such as tap water (28), certain traumatic manoeuvres, cleaning of the EAC, extraction of a cerumen plug, presence of a foreign body in the EAC or exposure to external radiotherapy (29-31).

2. LAND

The classic patient profile for this condition is the "elderly diabetic male", as originally described by Chandler (3). This can be explained by the altered immune defenses associated with age and diabetes.

2.1. Age

Several studies have concluded that advanced age is an important factor in the development of OEN. A series of 3 cases of OEN dating from 1984 included patients without underlying immunodeficiency conditions, the only major risk factor identified being advanced age. The ages of these patients were 87, 93 and 93 years (32).

An analysis of 8,300 patients hospitalized for SDO from 2002 to 2013 revealed that elderly patients (> 65 years of age) may have an increased risk of SDO complications and a poorer prognosis compared to younger patients. Specifically, this study reported that patients over the age of 65 had: more hospital procedures, longer hospitalizations, a greater likelihood of complications and higher in-hospital mortality (24).

Another study (Soudry et al) found that patients over 70 had a 5-year survival of 44%, while patients under 70 had a 5-year survival of 75% (33).

Compared with adults, OEN is even rarer in children. It has been noted in those with diabetes and other immunodepressing conditions such as immunoglobulin G (IgG) deficiency, immunoglobulin A (IgA) deficiency, leukemia, neutropenia, as well as after bone marrow transplantation. Overall, it is believed that children diagnosed with ESO have a more favorable prognosis than adults (34).

2.2. Diabetes

The risk factor most commonly reported in the literature for the development of ESO is diabetes mellitus (Table XXI), with an estimated 90-100% of ESO patients presenting with diabetes (18,35-37).

Table IV: Frequency of diabetes in necrotizing otitis externa in the literature

Study	Frequency of diabetes (%)
Azeez et al (37)	94
Peled et al (38)	94,3
Peled et al (39)	92,5
Byun et al (40)	82,1
Sylvester et al (24)	55,1
Sideris et al (25)	88,8
Yiğider et al (23)	96,1

Diabetes mellitus is thought to predispose patients to OEN due to microangiopathy, impaired wound healing and a diminished immune response. Indeed, microvascular lesions in diabetic patients, as well as defects in leukocyte phagocytosis and intracellular bacterial digestion, are factors favorable to the development of OEN.

In addition, variations in cerumen pH and a reduction in lytic components also favor bacterial growth in diabetic patients (41).

Although the association between OEN and diabetes is well established, our knowledge of the effects of diabetes duration and glycemic control on disease progression and outcome remains limited. Joshua et al (42) found that OEN patients with all mandatory parameters according to Friedman and Cohen's criteria had a higher incidence of diabetes, greater use of oral antidiabetic medication and a higher incidence of diabetes-related complications compared with OEN patients without all mandatory parameters.

Stern-Shavit et al (43) reported on patients from the same center and found that disease-specific mortality was correlated with and predicted by diabetes. Lee et al (44) reported that duration of diabetes was associated with uncontrolled OEN, but that HbA1c was not associated with OEN progression. Similarly, Loh et al (45) reported that diabetes severity, defined as HbA1c> 7%, was not associated with disease outcome.

Peled et al (38) showed that high levels of glycated hemoglobin (HbA1c) were associated with longer hospital stays in patients with OEN. Duration of diabetes and microalbuminuria were not correlated with the need for surgery and length of hospital stay. This may indicate that diabetic control at the time of disease onset, relative to total diabetic duration, plays a greater role in seeding bacteria in the surrounding bone, leading to severe disease requiring longer hospital treatment.

2.3. Other history

SDO can occur in a significant proportion of non-diabetic patients (9.1% of cases) (40), in which case it is mainly due to immune system dysfunction. Reasons for immunosuppression included hematological malignancy, solid cancer, history of organ transplantation, history of chemotherapy or radiotherapy, immune system deficiency (HIV), or use of chronic steroids or other immunosuppressants. These patients are more likely to develop external osteomyelitis due to their decreased resistance to infection, which allows the infection to spread around the external ear (41) (18).

These patients with immunosuppression due to HIV or other non-diabetic factors are more likely to develop OEN at a younger age than those with diabetes (46). In addition, people living with HIV have an increased risk of fungal infections and are likely to have a less favorable clinical course than diabetic patients (47).

OEN can also occur in immunocompetent patients (48,49):

- ❖ In some studies, hypertension and coronary insufficiency were often associated with SDO, since the latter electively affects the elderly (24) (50).
- ❖ In 2019, Bruschini et al (51) reported the case of a patient who, unlike most affected subjects, was neither diabetic nor immunosuppressed, but had been previously treated with radiotherapy in the head and neck region, 20 years before the onset of external osteomyelitis. Radiotherapy can induce a very slow process of bone necrosis, and bacterial infection could have invaded the necrotic tissue (18) (52).

3. DIAGNOSIS TIME

There is always a delay in diagnosis (Table XXII). In a review of the literature by Mahdyoun et al (53), the average delay was 70 days. This delay often corresponds to the first-line trial of local intra-auricular antibiotics, considered as a treatment for simple otitis externa, given the similarity of symptoms at an early stage (22).

Table V: Diagnosis times for patients with necrotizing otitis externa reported in the literature

Study	Number of cases	Diagnostic time (days)
Guevara et al (22)	22 cases	91
Glikson et al (27)	25 cases	42
Peled et al (28)	89 cases	33
Our series	116 cases	66

4. FUNCTIONAL SIGNS

The clinical picture of OEN is not very specific and is very similar to that of early-stage OE. Several studies have reported otalgia as the most common presenting symptom (27) (53). Signs peculiar to OEN compared with simple OE include disproportionate pain on examination and severe purulent otorrhea. The possibility of OEN should also be considered if otalgia persists for more than a month.

4.1 Otalgia

Otalgia is the most frequent (Table XXIII) and characteristic symptom of necrotizing otitis externa (22,27,39,50,54). This pain can be intense and stabbing, and is generally localized to the affected ear. It is aggravated by ear movement or pressure, and may even radiate to other parts of the head, neck or face. Pain is usually continuous, with a disabling nocturnal exacerbation resistant to the usual analgesics (55).

Table VI: Frequency of otalgia in the literature during necrotizing otitis externa

Study	Otalgia frequency (%)
Guevara et al (22)	100
Peled et al (39)	85,5
Takata et al (50)	96
Glikson et al (27)	100
Marina et al (54)	100

4.2 Otorrhea

Otorrhea is the 2nd most frequently described functional sign in the literature (22,37,50,54) (Table XXIV). In some studies, otorrhea was the most frequent reason for consultation (56-58). Its abundance is variable and tends to subside after a few days of antibiotic treatment. It is typically purulent and greenish (the color of pyocyanin produced by *Pseudomonas*), but can sometimes be bluish or even hemorrhagic. It is resistant to the usual antibiotic treatment of otitis externa.

Table VII: Frequency of otorrhea in the literature during necrotizing otitis externa

Study	Frequency of otorrhea (%)
Sekar et al (57)	100
Byun et al (58)	84,1
Marina et al (54)	71
Takata et al (50)	78

4.3. Headache

Headaches are generally located in the occipital and temporal regions (42, 48, 51). They are characterized by their intensity and resistance to first-line analgesics. According to Sekar (49), headache was present in 77.2% of patients, while Byun (50) reported 36.4%.

4.4 Hypoacusis

Hypoacusis is an inconsistent sign (Table XXV). It is often moderate and may be conductive, due to obstruction of the external auditory canal by granulations or edema, or sensorineural, due to aging or diabetes mellitus. It is confirmed by audiometry.

Table VIII: Frequency of hypoacusis in the literature during necrotizing otitis externa

Study	Frequency of hearing loss (%)
Lambor et al (59)	77,8
Azeez et al (37)	56,1
Singh et al (60)	25
Glikson et al (27)	16

4.5. Fever

Patients with NEO are generally apyretic. Indeed, the usual signs of infection are absent in necrotizing otitis externa (41). Patients may describe a fever, but the presence of fever is variable in the literature. For example, a systematic review by Mahdyoun, which included 48 studies, found that fever was documented in 5 studies with percentages ranging from 5% to 47% (53).
In other studies, fever was totally absent (27).

4.6. Tinnitus and vertigo

Tinnitus and vertigo have rarely been reported in the literature (9).

5. SEAT

In the literature, necrotizing otitis externa (NEO) is usually observed unilaterally (Table XXVI), but bilateral cases are not exceptional, with a frequency ranging from 11 to 64% (61). The majority of cases are right-sided (67% according to Bathokedeou's study (30), and 83.3% according to Balakrishnan's study (30,62).

Migirov (63) found a significant correlation between the lateralization of patients with OEN and the affected ear: among 34 right-handed patients, 70.6% had OEN on the right, compared with 29.4% on the left, while all left-handed patients had left-ear involvement ($p = 0.006$). These results underline the strong relationship between laterality and the ear affected in OEN. Migirov explained this relationship by hypothesizing that the development of OEN could be due to self-inflicted local trauma to the ear canal on the same side as the dominant hand.

Table IX: Percentage of unilaterality in the literature during necrotizing otitis externa

Study	Percentage of one-sidedness (%)
Bathokedeou et al (30)	100
Balakrishnan et al (62)	100
Guevara et al (22)	100
Peled et al (38)	97,7

6. PHYSICAL SIGNS

6.1 Inspection and palpation

ENT examination often reveals otorrhea (27,40,56,58), mastoid pain (64), TMJ pain (18,22,55,60), trismus (34,65), perichondritis (64). Cervical adenopathy is rarely observed on clinical examination.

6.2. Examination of cranial pairs

Nerve damage can appear early in the course of the disease, and is therefore one of the reasons for consultation. Usually, however, nerve damage occurs late in the course of the disease, and is a sign of its advanced stage. In fact, it is the most serious complication.

All cranial pairs should be examined systematically at the first consultation.

6.2.1. Facial paralysis

Involvement of the facial nerve is the most frequent and earliest, due to its proximity to the stylomastoid foramen (46,59) (Table XXVII). Pathophysiologically, facial paresis initially occurs due to mechanical compression of the VII nerve as it exits the skull at the stylomastoid foramen, and may progress to paralysis due to necrosis. Its frequency varies from study to study, ranging from 6 to 66% (24,44,50,53), with a tendency to decrease over time (27,38,39).

Involvement of the VII nerve is more frequent in children, reaching up to 53% (25). This is due to the facial nerve's closer proximity to the stylomastoid foramen.

This condition increases the risk of mortality (18,43,66).

Table X : Percentage of facial nerve involvement in the literature during necrotizing otitis externa

Study	Frequency of facial nerve damage (%)
Lee et al (44)	46,4
Takata et al (50)	21
Glikson et al (27)	8
Sylvester et al (24)	6,6

6.2.2. Involvement of other cranial pairs

Involvement of other cranial nerves is less frequent than that of the VII nerve, and is often associated with facial paralysis (44,64,66).

The nerves most frequently affected are: pneumogastric X, spinal XI, glossopharyngeal IX and hypoglossal XII (34,40,54,57). Cases of OEN involving the trigeminal V, abducens VI and optic II nerves were rarely reported (44,46). The olfactory I, oculomotor III and trochlear IV nerves appear to be unaffected in OEN (28).

Cranial nerve involvement is considered a prognostic factor in OEN, as it reflects the extent of the infection (31,67).

6.3. Otoscopy

Otoscopy during OEN may show an inflamed, more or less narrowed EAC, polyp, necrotic debris and/or granulation tissue at the floor of the EAC at the osteo-cartilaginous junction (18,34,46,68). The presence of granulation tissue is highly suggestive of OEN (Table XXVIII). However, this sign appears to be much rarer in HIV-infected patients and in children (28). Classically, the eardrum remains intact in OEN (31,69).

Table XI: Percentage of granulation tissue in the literature during necrotizing otitis externa

Study	Percentage of granulation fabric (%)
Peled et al (38)	72,5
Peled et al (39)	71
Byun et al (40)	78
Glikson et al (27)	96
Hasibi et al (56)	26,7
Stern Shavit et al (43)	75

CHAPTER 3:
FURTHER TESTS

1. BIOLOGY

1.1. Blood count

The CBC may be normal, or it may show hyperleukocytosis with PNN predominance (18,46).

1.2. CRP

There is little evidence of the sensitivity of CRP for the initial presentation of OEN, so negative results do not rule out the diagnosis (34). Although CRP is not specific to OEN, it may be useful for monitoring disease progression and response to antimicrobial therapy (46). Some studies have suggested that CRP levels help predict length of hospital stay and the need for antifungal therapy, thus helping to tailor management (70).

1.3. Blood glucose

OEN may be indicative of previously unrecognized diabetes, or it may lead to decompensation of existing diabetes. Therefore, it is recommended that close blood glucose monitoring be maintained during treatment of SDO in diabetic patients. In addition, people with no known history of diabetes should undergo a diabetes assessment after diagnosis of OEN (46).

2. MICROBIOLOGY

2.1. Local sampling

In the context of OEN, swabbing is a common method (50), but unreliable due to the high risk of contamination by commensal flora of the EAC. Syringe sampling of the ear discharge is preferable (71).

For cases of recurrent otitis externa, tissue sampling has proved to be of great value in selecting the appropriate antimicrobial treatment and ruling out other potential causes, such as malignancy or cholesteatoma (72).

The use of molecular methods, such as a polymerase chain reaction (PCR) test, favours pathogen detection in refractory culture-negative OEN (73,74).

Sampling should be carried out early in the course of treatment (46).

2.2. Bacteriology

Pseudomonas aeruginosa (P. aeruginosa) has long been reported as the most common causative agent of OEN (18,67,68). However, more recent studies suggest a decreasing prevalence *of P. aeruginosa* as the causative agent of OEN (34) and an increasing frequency of negative cultures (40). P. aeruginosa is an obligate aerobic Gram-negative germ, colonizing the EAC in a humid environment or after trauma. *P. aeruginosa* is not a normal component of the ear canal flora, even in diabetic patients, and its isolation must be considered abnormal and pathological.

In addition to *P. aeruginosa*, several other germs can cause OEN (28), including *Staphylococcus aureus, Klebsiella pneumoniae, Enterobacter,* coagulase-negative Staphylococci, *Escherichia coli, Proteus mirabilis* and *Enterococcus faecalis* (Table XXIX) .

Table XII: Percentage of different bacteria in necrotizing otitis externa according to the literature

Study	Percentage of *P. aeruginosa*	Other germs
Hobson et al (75)	45%	**Meti-sensitive Staphylococcus aureus:* 15%. **Multi-resistant Staphylococcus aureus:* 15%. * *Klebsiella pneumoniae:5% of the total* * *Acinetobacter:5%* * Enterococcus: 10%
Arsovic et al (12)	47%	* *Staphylococcus aureus: 10%.* * *Enterococcus: 3%.* * *Escherichia coli: 11%.* * *Proteus mirabilis: 3%.* *Streptococcus pyogenes:3%* * *Streptococcus pyogenes*
Sideris et al (25)	64%	*Staphylococcus:*19% * *Staphylococcus:*19% * *Staphylococcus:18* * Streptococcus*:* 6%.
Takata et al (50)	62%	* *Staphylococcus aureus:* 6%. **Enterobacter.spp:* 1%. * *Klebsiella.spp:2%* * *Proteus.spp:* 2% * *Escherichia coli:* 1%.

On the other hand, blood cultures have a limited role to play in OEN. Blood cultures are taken in the presence of general signs such as fever and chills.

2.3 Antibiotic sensitivity

Ciprofloxacin is the most widely used drug to treat OEN due to its low incidence of side effects, good tolerability and better penetration into cartilage. As observed in previous studies, *Pseudomonas* began to develop resistance to ciprofloxacin due to the widespread use of fluoroquinolones, both in systemic treatment and in topical ear drops. According to the literature, resistance to ciprofloxacin by *Pseudomonas* varies from 3% to 50% (40,50,57). This is because *Pseudomonas aeruginosa* is able to mutate its replication enzymes, which are the targets of fluoroquinolones, rendering them ineffective. It can also become resistant through the production of an insulating biofilm of polysaccharides preventing antibiotic diffusion (76).

This progressive increase in resistance over time can be avoided by limiting the use of fluoroquinolones in outpatient benign otitis externa.

According to the literature, the main germs isolated are sensitive to amikacin, cefapérazone-sulbactam and piperacillin. This shows how antibiotic resistance has prompted the use of higher-end antibiotics to treat this infection (57).

2.4. Mycology

In the literature, mycological studies are often carried out in patients already on antibiotics (77). A fungal cause is suspected if anti-pyocyanic antibiotics fail. This stipulates that OENs are considered to be bacterial in origin, hence the delay in diagnosis and treatment of fungal OENs. This is the main pejorative factor in mycotic OEN (40).

In our study, the 2 fungi most frequently isolated *in* the literature were *Candida.spp* and *Aspergillus.spp* (34,50), with *Aspergillus* predominating (31,47,56,78). The most frequent species was *Aspergillus flavus*, and for *Candida*, the most frequent species was *Candida albicans* (79).

2.5. Sensitivity to antifungal agents

Sensitivity to antifungal agents was debated in several studies. *Aspergillus*, the fungus most responsible for OEN, is generally sensitive to voriconazole (79). Some studies found voriconazole and ketoconazole to be the most effective antifungal agents, particularly against *Aspergillus niger* and *Candida albicans* (80). Others have shown caspofungin to be highly active against *Aspergillus* and *Candida* isolates (81).

Candida, especially *Candida albicans*, is highly sensitive to fluconazole (79), with some resistance observed in a few cases (82).

3. IMAGING DATA

Imaging plays an important role, not only in the positive diagnosis of OEN, but also in determining the extent of infection and assessing response to treatment.

The most commonly used imaging modalities are computed tomography (CT), magnetic resonance imaging (MRI), radionuclides and fluorodeoxyglucose positron emission tomography (FDG PET/CT) (49).

Several studies have compared the superiority of different imaging techniques, while others have examined the multifaceted approach and optimal use of specific imaging modalities to achieve the best results.

3.1 Rock computed tomography (CT)

Computed tomography (CT) is ideal for assessing bone erosion, hence its value in the initial diagnosis of OEN (28). It can be performed with or without contrast injection. Bone and parenchymal window exploration with axial and coronal reconstructions is required.

3.1.1. Realization

In the literature, CT scans of the rock were performed in 60-100% of cases (39,45,83,84).

3.1.2. Results

In cases of OEN, CT of the rocks can show involvement of the external auditory canal, mastoid, temporomandibular joint and skull base. Soft tissue involvement, such as filling of the middle ear and mastoid, as well as involvement of the nasopharynx, can also be observed by CT. These findings also have prognostic value, as demonstrated by several studies (85,86).

Osteolysis, CAE filling and mastoid cells are the main lesions detected on CT (46,85) (Table XXX).

Table XIII: CT scan data for necrotizing otitis externa

	Peled (39)	Salaheddine (87)	Peled (83)
Osteolysis (%)	29,8	100	-
CAE filling (%)	61,4	100	60
Mastoid cell filling (%)	94,6	80	65
Filling of tympanic cavity (%)	35	-	50
Peri-auricular soft tissue involvement (%)	-	15	-
TMJ arthritis (%)	-	10	5
Skull base osteitis (%)	-	-	10

*CAE: external auditory canal *ATM: temporomandibular joint

3.1.3. Benefits

Because bone erosion distinguishes malignant otitis externa from otitis externa, computed tomography (CT) is the most commonly used imaging modality for the 1st-line diagnosis of OEN and skull base osteitis (28,88).

CT imaging is often considered a relatively easy and rapid method of obtaining an overview of the mastoid region. The strength of this modality lies in the assessment of bone erosion and demineralization (88). Thus, CT allows better identification of posterior spread of OEN, probably because the pattern of posterior spread is based solely on cortical destruction of the mastoid of the temporal bone, a structure that cannot be optimally assessed by MRI (89). CT allows analysis of skull-base bone density and soft-tissue abscess formation. It also assesses involvement of the mastoid, temporomandibular joint, infratemporal fossa, nasopharynx, petrous apex and carotid canal. (90).

3.1.4. Limits

Although CT is the imaging modality of choice for the treatment of OEN, it does have its limitations. Osteolysis, although a frequent finding in OEN, is not specific to this condition. It can also be associated with many other conditions, such as benign or malignant tumors or congenital lesions. Moreover, CT cannot differentiate between an inflammatory and a neoplastic cause (91).

On the other hand, bone erosion is not evident on CT until around 30% of the bone is demineralized. Consequently, early bone erosion may not be detectable on CT, leading to delays in diagnosis (41). High false-negative rates have been described in the literature, up to 41% (89,92). It is also inadequate for detecting endocranial extension or soft-tissue involvement (88). It is also unsuitable for therapeutic follow-up (93). Indeed, several studies have reported that CT findings do not correlate with clinical evolution (28).

3.2. Bone scintigraphy

This is a key examination, usually showing hyperfixation in the rock (31). Two radioelements can be used: technetium-99m and gallium-67.

3.2.1. Technetium-99m scintigraphy

3.2.1.1. Technique

Technetium-99m scintigraphy (^{99m} Tc) involves injecting methylene diphosphonate labeled with ^{99m} Tc and taking a series of early (at 5 minutes), late (at 4 hours) and very late (at 24 hours) images using a gamma camera.

Technetium 99m binds to hydroxyapatite crystals, with more intense fixation (hyperfixation) in areas of increased osteoblastic activity. In the case of OENs, this examination reveals infection-induced bone destruction through hyperfixation.

3.2.1.2. Benefits

Scintigraphy has excellent sensitivity (31). In a recent meta-analysis, the overall sensitivity of technetium (^{99m} Tc) was 96.99% (94). Even a 10% increase in osteoblastic activity can be detected (88), enabling early diagnosis. What's more, the technique is inexpensive and readily available (88).

3.2.1.3. Limits

Bone scintigraphy, although sensitive, is not specific (31), as it also shows increased fixation in any condition of high bone turnover, for example in the postoperative state or in malignancy with bone involvement (88).

It is also unsuitable for monitoring the progress of resolution, as bone remodelling persists for several months after clinical healing, and so scintigraphy will continue to give positive results (90).

To overcome this lack of specificity, some authors have recommended the use of the technetium-linked murine monoclonal antibody (^{99m} Tc sulesomab), approved for osteomyelitis imaging, which provides an accurate reflection of disease activity and response to treatment (95).

Since ^{99m}Tc scintigraphy also lacks anatomical precision, combining this radionuclide with single-photon emission computed tomography (SPECT) as well as with CT or MRI offers more accurate and informative imaging (46,93).

3.2.2. Gallium scintigraphy 67

3.2.2.1. Technique

An initial gallium 67 (Ga67) scintigraphy is indicated during the initial work-up of OEN. The radioisotope is incorporated into actively dividing bacteria and granulocytes, so serial imaging over a period of time could be used to determine the duration of antibiotic treatment and monitor response to therapy (31).

3.2.2.2. Benefits

Gallium-67 scintigraphy has excellent sensitivity, with 93.78% reported in the literature (94).

When osteomyelitis is active, both ^{99m} Tc and 67Ga scans are positive, but when osteomyelitis is inactive, the 67Ga scan is negative. It can therefore be used to assess the efficacy of treatment for malignant otitis externa (41). Its negativity is considered a major criterion for cure. Antibiotics can then be discontinued if the tomographic images have normalized on gallium scintigraphy (95).

3.2.2.3. Limits

Gallium 67 scintigraphy, like ^{99m}Tc, is sensitive but non-specific (31). It does not differentiate between infectious and tumoral origins.

Although several studies have reported that gallium scintigraphy can be used to monitor disease activity, others have noted that normal scans can be observed in patients with recurrent disease (28). Moreover, this technique provides little anatomical detail and low resolution, underlining the importance of integrating it with the information provided by CT, MRI (95), or single-photon emission computed tomography (SPECT) (28).

The high cost and difficulty of access to gallium bone scintigraphy, as well as its high radiation exposure, remain major problems limiting the feasibility of this exploration in the radiological assessment of OEN (96).

3.3 Magnetic resonance imaging (MRI)

3.3.1. Benefits

By comparing MRI with CT:

- ❖ MRI allows early diagnosis before the appearance of bone erosion on CT (28).

- Thanks to its excellent resolution, MRI is the examination of choice for studying the extension of lesions to the soft tissues and bone marrow. It can detect infiltration of intracranial and lateropharyngeal spaces, nerve foramen, dura mater and skull base. Thus, MRI is useful for determining prognosis by showing extension (extension in more than one direction is associated with a worse prognosis) and looking for local complications such as venous thrombosis (28,46,89,93).
- MRI is the examination of choice for detecting cranial nerve damage, particularly to nerves VII and VIII (46,93).
- MRI can be used to distinguish skull base osteomyelitis, secondary to malignant otitis externa, from nasopharyngeal carcinoma (97).

3.3.2. Limits

- MRI is more expensive than CT and less accessible.
- MRI is not recommended for therapeutic follow-up of patients with OEN, as the morphological appearance of lesions remains unchanged for a long time (46,93).
- MRI is less specific than it is sensitive: it can give false negatives in the early stages of the disease, and can sometimes confuse an infectious origin with tumor involvement (41).

3.4. Positron emission tomography/computed tomography (PET/CT)

Positron emission tomography combined with CT can detect metabolically active tissue, making it an ideal test for identifying and monitoring malignancies or localized infections (46). It has a better specificity than MRI or CT alone (91%) and a sensitivity of 96% (86).

18F-FDG-PET/CT is described as a reliable imaging modality for diagnosis, localization of disease and decision making regarding discontinuation of treatment for OEN. Some studies have considered PET/CT as the imaging modality of choice for the initial diagnosis and follow-up of patients with OEN due to its advantages in terms of sensitivity, specificity, cost and radiation exposure (86,96).

In certain situations, PET/CT may not differentiate OEN from temporal bone tumors (86).

4. ANATOMOPATHOLOGY

Anatomopathological study of ear samples collected by biopsy of the CAE is not systematic. It is reserved for patients who have not responded to antibiotic therapy or in whom cultures are negative without clinical improvement. It is the only definitive method for distinguishing OEN from tumour involvement (28).

Mycotic SDO can also be confirmed by the presence of mycelial filaments in granulation tissue with a positive culture (92).

Biopsy of the external auditory canal may reveal ulceration and loss of epithelium, with bacteria and inflammation extending into the dense fibrous tissue. In areas where the epithelium remains intact, reactive changes may range from mild hyperplasia to pseudoepitheliomatous hyperplasia. Acute and chronic inflammation, including abscess formation, is common. In biopsy samples taken from the cartilage duct, inflammation often extends into the apopilosebaceous units (46).

CHAPTER 4:
POSITIVE DIAGNOSIS

1. POSITIVE DIAGNOSIS OF NECROTIZING OTITIS EXTERNA

The diagnosis of OEN requires a strong index of suspicion based on several criteria, such as a comprehensive medical history, clinical signs, underlying conditions likely to compromise the immune system, biological markers such as an increase in CRP, the presence of certain bacteriological or fungal pathogens found and radiological evidence with or without bone erosion in the external auditory canal and infratemporal fossa (93).

At present, there is no universally acceptable diagnostic criterion for SDO (31). In a recent systematic review (50) including 51 articles: 18% used the case definition proposed by Cohen and Friedman (98) and 6% used a modified definition. A minority (22%) included risk factors in their case definition, notably diabetes or immunodeficiency. The most common case definition criterion was "failure of symptoms to improve with outpatient treatment" (80%).

In the literature, certain diagnostic criteria were established by:

- Corey (99) published in 1985:
  - Persistent external otitis.
  - Granulation tissue in the external auditory canal.
  - Radiological evidence of mastoiditis or osteomyelitis of the skull base.
  - Cranial nerve paralysis.
  - *Pseudomonas* in bacteriological sampling.

This study (99) also has prognostic value, identifying 3 stages of OEN.

- Cohen (98) in 1987 divided the diagnostic criteria into major criteria whose presence is mandatory and minor criteria (Table XXXI).

Table XIV: Cohen's diagnostic criteria for necrotizing otitis externa

Major criteria	Minor criteria
• Pain	• *Pseudomonas* in the sample
• Exudate	• Positive X-ray including CT scan
• Edema	• Diabetes
• Granulation tissues	• Damage to the cranial pairs
• Microabscesses confirmed by surgery	• A debilitated terrain
• Positive technetium-99m scan	• Elderly

On the other hand, some studies have pointed to the value of making an early diagnosis of SDO before all the major criteria have been met, to guarantee a better prognosis (28).

- Levenson (100) in 1991 combined the following 7 criteria:
  - Refractory otitis externa.
  - Severe otalgia.
  - A purulent exudate.
  - The presence of granulation tissue in the floor of the EAC.
  - The presence of *Pseudomonas aeruginosa* in the exudate culture.
  - A particular condition (elderly, diabetic or immunocompromised patient).
  - Petrous fixation on late-stage ^{99m} Tc scintigraphy.

Table XXXII illustrates the relative frequency of the different LEVENSON diagnostic criteria in different series in the literature.

Table XV: LEVENSON diagnostic criteria

	Lambor et al. (59)	Emin Karmen et al. (69)	Bruno et al. (101)	Our study
Refractory otitis externa	100%	100%	100%	100%
Severe earache	100%	100%	100%	88,8%
Purulent exudate	81,5%	100%	72,7%	67%
Granulation fabric	92,6%	100%	100%	26,7%
Presence of *Pseudomonas*	41,7%	90%	81.8%	50%
Private lot	100%	100%	100%	89,6%
Positive scintigraphy	-	40%	27,2%	18,9%

2. CLASSIFICATION OF NECROTIZING OTITIS EXTERNA

In the literature, there are 3 ancient classifications based on anatomoclinical and radiological data to define the severity of involvement.

- ❖ Classification by COREY (99) (Table XXXIII):

Table XVI: COREY 1985 classification

Stage I	Infection of the soft and bony tissues of the external auditory canal without affecting the cranial pairs.
Stage II	Involvement of the cranial pairs: 1-Facial nerve damage 2-Damage to other cranial pairs.
Stage III	Serious complications: 1-Meningitis; 2-Empyema of the epidural ; 3-Subdural emphysema; 4-abcessed brain

❖ LEVENSON classification (100) (Table XXXIV):

Table XVII: LEVENSON classification

Stage I: Necrotizing external pre-otitis	Presence of one of these criteria (diabetic, elderly or immunocompromised patient, otitis externa with intense otalgia especially at night, purulent otorrhea with *Pseudomonas aeruginosa*, dragging otitis externa, granulation tissue in the EAC)
Stage II: Limited OEN	Stage I with positive ^{99m}Tc scintigraphy
Stage III: Central OEN	Stage II with involvement of the TMJ, skull base, parapharyngeal spaces, infratemporal fossa and/or cranial nerve paralysis.

TMJ: temporomandibular joint

❖ Classification by THAKAR 1996 (102) (Table XXXV):

Table XVIII: THAKAR classification

Stage I	Necrotizing otitis externa (persistent ear pain, bare bone at the EAC, absence of facial paralysis)
Stage II	Limited skull base osteomyelitis (facial nerve damage)
Stage III	Extensive skull base osteomyelitis (involvement of jugular foramen, intracranial extension).

EAC: external auditory meatus

CHAPTER 5:
PROGNOSIS AND SPECIAL FORMS

1. PROGNOSIS

Several factors are associated with a poor prognosis in patients with OEN: such as facial nerve palsy, fungal etiology of OEN, relapse of OEN, recourse to surgery and major radiological findings (bone erosion, intracranial or oropharyngeal involvement on CT or MRI) suggesting that the infection has crossed its anatomical boundaries and spread to adjacent tissue compartments (12,66). On the other hand, association with signs of intracranial infection, such as meningitis, abscess formation or septic venous thrombosis, are often fatal and represent a late stage of OEN (34).

Several studies have evaluated the use of facial nerve palsy as a prognostic indicator. Facial nerve involvement has been suggested as an unfavorable prognostic indicator of OEN, indicating advanced disease (34,43). However, some research has found no significant difference in survival between patients with facial nerve palsy and those without (103). Certain comorbidities can worsen the prognosis of SDO and prolong the duration of hospitalization, such as weight loss, diabetes with chronic complications, congestive heart failure, coagulopathy, liver disease and aging with age over 70 (13,43,103).

2. SPECIAL FORMS

2.1. Fungal necrotizing otitis externa

Mycotic involvement is currently increasingly common, especially in immunocompromised subjects of advanced age, as in our series, where the mean age of patients with fungal ENT was 68.8±10.8 years, whereas in the case of bacterial ENT the mean age was 60 ± 15 years.

Fungal OEN is characterized by mastoid and middle ear involvement, more frequent facial nerve involvement, a guarded prognosis and higher mortality (Table XXXVI).

Table XIX: Comparison between fungal and bacterial necrotizing otitis externa

	OEN Bacterial	**OEN Fungal**
Bilaterality (8)	10%	33%
Duration of symptoms before hospitalization (56)	9-12 weeks	>12 weeks
Facial paralysis (8) (56)	14% 17,3%	55% 28,7%
Imaging (8)	-	Greater mastoid and middle ear involvement
Prognosis (34)	-	More serious
Treatment (47.79)	-	Greater use of surgery and HBOT
Positive bacterial culture on presentation (8)	75%	33%
Persistent SDO (8)	12%	89%

NEO: necrotizing otitis externa HBOT: hyperbaric oxygen therapy

2.2 Necrotizing otitis externa in children

OEN is rare in children (46). It mainly affects children with diabetes and/or other immunodeficiency conditions, including IgG deficiency, IgA deficiency or bone marrow transplantation. Leukemia, neutropenia and anemia are also risk factors for ESO in children (28,34).

In children, OEN is more frequently complicated by facial paralysis, which may even inaugurate the disease. This predisposition has been attributed to the facial nerve's closer proximity to the stylomastoid foramen (34).

Pediatric patients are more symptomatic on initial examination (24). The prognosis of OEN is better than in adults, with shorter hospital stays, lower total hospital costs and less need for debridement, ear biopsy or hyperbaric oxygen therapy (24).

2.3 Necrotizing otitis externa in the immunocompromised

OEN has also been described in various contexts of immunosuppression other than diabetes: such as retroviral infection (HIV), neoplasia, hematologic malignancy, immunosuppressive therapy or prolonged corticosteroid therapy (28,46). These patients develop OEN at an earlier age than diabetics. In the setting of HIV retroviral infection, patients present a higher risk of fungal infections, especially to *Aspergillus*.spp. The prognosis is less favorable than in diabetic patients. In addition, they may lack granulation tissue in the EAC on otoscopy (46,47).

Other rarer germs may be isolated from patients with immunosuppression due to HIV or other non-diabetic factors, such as: *Scedosporium apiospermum, Pseudallescheria boydii, Candida ciferrii, Candida orthopsilosis and Malassezia sympodialis* (28).

2.4. Immunocompetent form

Although malignant otitis externa is frequently observed in elderly or immunocompromised diabetic patients, it can be seen in immunocompetent subjects. Symptomatology is the same as in diabetic subjects (25,49).

2.5. Bilateral form

A few cases of bilateral OEN have been published in the world literature. This highlights the power of propagation and the damage that can be caused by OEN (53). In our study, 12 cases (10.3%) were bilateral.

CHAPTER 6:
DIFFERENTIAL DIAGNOSIS

The differential diagnosis of OEN includes several entities: otitis externa, mastoiditis, Paget's disease, keratosis obturans, seborrheic dermatitis, ear canal carcinoma, cholesteatoma, suppurative labyrinthitis, otitis media and perichondritis (31,34,46).

1. SIMPLE EXTERNAL OTITIS

Otitis externa (OE) is an infection leading to inflammation of the EAC. OEN may be clinically indistinguishable from simple OE at the onset of the disease. It is more common in children and shares the same risk factors as OEN: swimming or other outdoor water exposure, ear trauma due to excessive cleaning or scratching, and the use of ear devices such as earplugs or hearing aids. The picture is identical to that of OEN: otalgia, otorrhea, deafness. On otoscopy, the ear canal may be partially or completely obstructed by debris or purulent discharge, but the tympanic membrane should appear normal if visualized (as in OEN). In addition, the EAC usually appears erythematous and inflamed. In otitis externa, otalgia is sensitive to 1[er] analgesics, and evolution is often favorable after 7 days of usual treatment (34).

2. MASTOIDITIS

Necrotizing otitis externa can also be confused with mastoiditis in the paediatric population. Mastoiditis occurs most frequently in children. The majority of cases involve patients under 2 years of age (104). The most common symptoms included malaise, abnormal tympanic membrane, post-auricular erythema, pinna tenderness and/or protrusion, fever, narrowing of the EAC, ear pain and otorrhea (34). Mastoiditis can be diagnosed using computed tomography (CT) (105).

3. TUBERCULOUS OTITIS EXTERNA

Tuberculous otitis externa, a rare localization of extra-pulmonary tuberculosis, can present as a chronic, purulent infection of the middle ear and, to a lesser degree, the outer ear (106). It is often characterized by treatment-resistant otorrhea, and can lead to complications such as facial nerve paralysis and progressive hearing loss. Extracranial tuberculosis, mainly of the lungs, is frequently present. Diagnosis is based on direct culture of *Mycobacterium tuberculosis* (107).

4. CHOLESTEATOMATOUS OTITIS MEDIA

Cholesteatomatous otitis media and necrotizing otitis externa share many similarities. Both conditions can present with otalgia, otorrhea and hearing loss. However, otoscopic examination under a microscope can usually distinguish them by showing the presence of a cholesteatomatous matrix (108). The nature of the bone erosion may be a key factor in distinguishing these conditions (109). Cholesteatomatous otitis, like OEN, predominates in elderly subjects, with a mean age of 58 ± 17.9 years. It may occur in children, with the possibility of congenital pathogenesis and other associated factors such as ventilation tube insertion (108,110).

5. WEGENER'S GRANULOMATOSIS

Wegener's granulomatosis can affect the outer ear, manifesting as a wide range of head and neck symptoms and destruction of the temporal bone with involvement of the cranial pairs (111). Histological examination reveals a necrotizing vasculitis in favor of Wegener's granulomatosis (112).

6. SQUAMOUS CELL CARCINOMA

Carcinoma of the temporal bone may also present as otalgia and otorrhea. Since radiological studies cannot differentiate tumor from necrotizing infection, biopsy is the only definitive method of distinguishing these two entities. The association of these 2 pathologies has been reported in the literature (28). Some authors have pointed out the importance of suspecting a neoplastic process in the event of a poor therapeutic response, with the indispensable recourse to an EAC biopsy to rectify the diagnosis (31).

7. GIANT CELL TUMORS OF THE SKULL BASE

Symptomatology in these tumors may be similar to that of necrotizing otitis externa (113).

8. MIDDLE EAR ASPERGILLOMA

Aspergilloma of the middle ear can mimic necrotizing otitis externa. Both may present with otalgia, otorrhea, hypoacusis, and may involve the facial nerve (114). Anatomopathological examination can help to correct the diagnosis.

CHAPTER 7:
PROCESSING

The management of OEN has undergone a major revolution since its first descriptions, with the evolution of recently developed effective antimicrobial drugs and a multidisciplinary approach to treatment. Before the era of antibiotics active against *Pseudomonas aeruginosa*, the outcome of the disease was fatal in the majority of cases.

Strict glycemic control, correction of electrolyte imbalances, improved immunity, auricular hygiene, hyperbaric oxygen therapy and prolonged systemic and ototopic antimicrobial therapy, have become crucial in the effective treatment of OEN (20,31).

Surgery is considered when non-surgical treatments have proved ineffective, and involves procedures such as local debridement, abscess drainage or removal of bone sequestration (46).

1. LAND TREATMENT

Treating the terrain requires a multidisciplinary approach. Therefore, we must establish:

- Diabetes management consisting of insulin therapy, strict and adequate glycemic control via HbA1c measurement and serial blood glucose monitoring (26,57,84,115).
- Improved immunocompetence (116).

2. ANTIBIOTICS

2.1. Choices and associations

Early and appropriate antibiotic therapy can prevent bone destruction and subsequent spread of OEN to intracranial structures. Cultures of the external auditory canal (EAC) drainage should be obtained prior to antimicrobial therapy, as culture results will guide the choice of molecule (34,117).

Table XXXVII summarizes the numerous associations cited in the literature.

Table XX: Antibiotic combinations found in the literature.

Study	Number of cases	Antibiotic therapy
Hariga et al (120)	19 cases	Ceftazidime+Gentamycin:3cases. Ofloxacin+Gentamycin:3cases. Ofloxacin+Ceftazidime: 13 cases.
C. Pulcini et al (121)	32 cases	Ceftazidime+ ciprofloxacin: 27 cases. Fosfomycin (IV) + ceftazidime: 1 case. Piperacillin-tazobactam +fosfomycin (IV): 1 case. Ceftazidime: 2 cases. Clindamycin+ciprofloxacin: 1 case.
S. Chabbret et al (76)	32 cases	Ciprofloxacin+ ceftazidime: 25 cases. Meropenem+fosfomycin: 1 case. Piperacillin+tazobactam+ciprofloxacin: 3 cases. Teicoplanin+clindamycin: 1 case. Pristinamycin+ciprofloxacin+ceftazidime: 1 case. Cloxacillin+ciprofloxacin: 1 case.
Carlton et al (117)	12 cases	Cefepime + Ciprofloxacin: 4 cases. Vancomycin+ Cefepime+ Levofloxacin: 1case. Piperacillin/tazobactam+ Cefepime or Ceftazidime: 2 cases. Meropenem +Ciprofloxacin: 2 cases. Aztreonam: 1 case. Vancomycin + Meropenem: 1 case. Piperacillin/tazobactam+ Cefepime+ Ciprofloxacin: 1case.

Antipseudomonas antimicrobials are the cornerstone of OEN treatment (28). Several authors have demonstrated the value of fluoroquinolones in the treatment of *Pseudomonas* ESO, which has dramatically improved the prognosis of this condition (27,28,117). In addition to their excellent activity against *P. Aeruginosa*, fluoroquinolones have a bone and cartilage concentration seven times higher than serum and low renal toxicity, given the precarious state of renal function in diabetics, making them well suited to OEN (31,117). Ciprofloxacin is the most widely used molecule. Long-term monotherapy of 6 to 8 weeks with oral ciprofloxacin (750 mg twice daily) may be indicated as initial antibiotic therapy. However, ciprofloxacin has limited coverage against gram-positive bacteria and does not cover MRSA (methicillin-resistant *Staphylococcus aureus*) (34).

In addition, more recent studies have shown the emergence of more and more fluoroquinolone-resistant strains *of Pseudomonas* (32,45). This resistance varies considerably according to clinical context, with rates reaching 30-33% in some settings (34,118). Overuse of fluoroquinolones in uncomplicated otitis and ENT and/or upper respiratory infections, a previous stay in intensive care, diabetes mellitus and nosocomial residence are risk factors for fluoroquinolone-resistant *P. aeruginosa* (34,118,119).

If resistance to fluoroquinolones is suspected, combinations with other agents with *antipseudomonas* activity should be prescribed, such as piperacillin-tazobactam, ceftazidime, cefepime and meropenem (118).

Currently, the most widely recommended treatment protocol in the literature is a parenteral combination of a fluoroquinolone and a 3rd generation cephalosporin (C3G), followed by an oral fluoroquinolone (20,53,103,117,120).

The combination of imipenem and ciprofloxacin is also indicated for the treatment of OEN in cases of C3G resistance due to the production of a cephalosporinase, which results in resistance to all beta-lactams tested, with the exception of imipenem (36).

In addition to the germ's resistance profile, the choice of antibiotic therapy depends on the severity of the condition:

- For immunocompetent patients with uncomplicated necrotizing otitis externa (28):
  - ➔ Intravenous (IV) ciprofloxacin as monotherapy (in adults: 400 mg IV 3 times a day, in children: 20 to 30 mg/kg per day IV divided every 12 hours, max 800 mg/day).
  - ➔ Oral follow-up with ciprofloxacin (adults: 750 mg twice daily, children: 20 to 30 mg/kg daily, divided every 12 hours, max. 1500 mg/day).
- For patients with advanced necrotizing otitis externa (significant bone erosion, multiple cranial neuropathies) or immunosuppressed conditions, or when the local rate of fluoroquinolone resistance in Pseudomonas is very high (28):
  - ➢ Initial dual therapy with ciprofloxacin plus an antipseudomonas beta-lactam:
    - ✓ Piperacillin:
      - Adults: 3 g IV *6/day or 4 g IV *4/day.
      - Children: 50 to 75 mg/kg IV every four to six hours (do not exceed 4 g per dose or 24 g per day).
    - ✓ Piperacillin-tazobactam:
      - Adults: 4 g/500mg IV *4/day.

- Children ≤40 kg: 300 mg/kg of piperacillin per day IV divided over 3 doses (do not exceed 16 g per day of piperacillin component).
- Children >40 kg: 3 g every six hours or 4 g every six to eight hours.

✓ Ceftazidime:
- Adults: 2 g IV *3/day.
- Children: 100 to 150 mg/kg per day IV divided every eight hours (do not exceed 6 g per day).

✓ Cefepime:
- Adults: 2 g IV *2/day (in severe *P. aeruginosa* infections, we can give 2g*3/day).
- Children: 50 mg/kg IV every eight hours (not to exceed 2 g per dose).

✓ Meropenem:
- Adults: 2 g IV *3/day.
- Children: 60 mg/kg/day IV divided every eight hours (not to exceed 3 g per day), in case of intracranial extension: 120 mg/kg/day IV divided every eight hours (not to exceed 6 g per day).

➢ Oral relay with ciprofloxacin.

❖ For patients with evidence of sepsis, systemic infection or intracranial spread, broad-spectrum antimicrobial coverage is warranted (122,123):

➢ Vancomycin (30 mg/kg IV) + cefepime or ceftazidime or meropenem.

➢ If intracranial abscess is suspected: metronidazole should be added to the above-mentioned treatment regimen.

2.2. Duration of treatment

Duration of treatment depends on response to therapy. Patients should be reassessed every 4 to 6 weeks during treatment with a Ga-67 scan. Antibiotic therapy should be discontinued one week after a normal Ga-67 scan, provided that inflammatory markers have also normalized. Even after resolution of the infection, high-risk patients should undergo periodic reassessment for one year, as recurrences may occur (46).

According to the literature, a minimum duration of antibiotic therapy of 4 to 8 weeks is recommended (20,28,31,124). This recommendation is based on the time required for bone vascular reconstruction, which takes around 3 to 4 weeks (41).

3. ANTIFUNGALS

3.1 Choice of antifungals

For patients with HIV, severe immunosuppression or antibiotic treatment failure, fungal SDO should be suspected and the patient prescribed an empirical antifungal agent (41).

Before the advent of new antifungal agents such as fluconazole and voriconazole, the treatment of ESO was based on amphotericin B, followed by itraconazole in the majority of cases (34,50,56).

Over the years, therapeutic strategies have evolved considerably. Patients are treated according to the fungus isolated, its sensitivity to antifungal agents and the molecules available (27,125,126). Fluconazole and voriconazole are better tolerated than amphotericin B, with good oral bioavailability and bone diffusion, making them the first-line treatment for fungal OEN. Caspofungin is rarely used (47,127,128).

3.1.1. Necrotizing candidous otitis externa

Candida is frequently sensitive to all triazole derivatives. For *Candida-induced* OEN, fluconazole can be prescribed as first-line treatment (79), except for *Candida krusei*, which is naturally resistant, and *Candida glabrata*, whose sensitivity to fluconazole is diminished. Voriconazole is also effective, and even superior to fluconazole (59,77).

3.1.2. Aspergillosis necrotizing otitis externa

In the case of *Aspergillus* OEN, prolonged treatment with voriconazole may be the therapy of choice (28,47,129). Alternative therapy with liposomal amphotericin B may be prescribed. Voriconazole proved superior to amphotericin B in a randomized controlled trial in patients with other types of invasive *Aspergillus* infections (mainly pulmonary) (28). Isavuconazole, a new triazole shown to be non-inferior to voriconazole in the treatment of invasive *Aspergillus* infections, may also be an option for treating malignant *Aspergillus* otitis externa (130).

3.2. Duration of antifungal treatment

The authors recommend antifungal treatment for a minimum of 2 to 3 months (56,78,79,131).

4. LOCAL TREATMENT AND CARE

4.1. Local care

The importance of local care in the treatment of OEN has been emphasized by several authors in the literature (120).

This treatment includes (132):

- Aspiration of purulent secretions.
- Local debridement of granulation tissue.
- Removal of bone or cartilage sequestration where present.
- Drainage of any abscess.

Good calibration of the external auditory canal using the colymicin-soaked pope wick.

These treatments are essential to dry out the ear, relieve pain and ensure better diffusion of local antibiotics.

4.2. Local antibiotic therapy

In a recent review, local antibiotic therapy was used in 51% of cases (50). The most commonly used ear drops are ofloxacin, ciprofloxacin/dexamethasone and polymyxin B/neomycin/hydrocortisone (46). However, the efficacy of this local antibiotic therapy remains ambiguous. Many authors advocate its use and consider it one of the mainstays in the management of OEN (27), while others assert that these preparations modify the bacterial flora of the ACE, decrease the rate of positive cultures and create antibiotic resistance without adding any significant benefit (28,34,46). Further work on the efficacy of local antibiotic therapy is therefore required (84).

In our study, topical antibiotics were prescribed to 50 patients (43.1%).

4.3. Local corticosteroid therapy

Ototopic corticoids have an anti-inflammatory and analgesic action in the treatment of simple otitis externa (133). However, some authors have suggested the potential risk of fungal OEN and otomycosis following intra-auricular instillation of corticosteroids (134,135).

5. HYPERBARIC OXYGEN THERAPY

5.1 Indications

Several authors have indicated the use of hyperbaric oxygen therapy (HBOT) in the treatment of various infectious lesions as an adjuvant therapy to antibiotics (136). In the case of OEN, HBOT was reported to be a valuable adjunct to antibiotics, enabling surgery to be deferred and the duration of antibiotic treatment reduced. It should be considered in advanced forms with significant skull base involvement and intracranial extension, and in cases of recurrence (28,50,58,137). Some authors have indicated HBOT in cases where well-managed medical treatment has failed for two or three weeks (138). However, numerous studies show no additional benefit from its use as an adjuvant to medical or surgical therapy (28,46,136).

5.2. Mechanism of action

HBOT provides tissue hyperoxia, which promotes healing and scarring of lesions (34). Indeed, it can induce vasoconstriction, reduce CAE edema, and increase the portion of oxygen dissolved in the blood to improve oxygenation of poorly vascularized and necrotic areas. HBOT has a healing effect by increasing angiogenesis and stimulating fibroblasts to form collagen. It also potentiates the bactericidal activity of leukocytes by stimulating phagocytosis (41). Moreover, HBOT even enhances the antibacterial efficacy of certain antibiotics, such as aminoglycosides (139).

5.3. Complications

HBOT can lead to complications of varying severity (139):

- ❖ The most common complication is reversible progressive myopia due to corneal deformation.
- ❖ Barotrauma of the sinuses and middle ear has been described, and can be prevented by pressure equalization techniques.
- ❖ Pulmonary barotrauma and pneumothorax are extremely rare.
- ❖ Gas embolisms are exceptional when preventive measures are taken.
  - ➔ These complications can be prevented by taking breaks during the hyperbaric oxygen therapy session.

6. SURGERY

Prior to advances in antibiotic therapy, extensive surgery to remove all infected tissue was the ideal treatment for malignant otitis externa. This involved local debridement with/without deep-tissue biopsy, mastoidectomy, facial nerve decompression and petrosectomy (43,83).

In the literature (140,44,46,66,73), surgery was indicated in the event of..:

- ❖ Non-response to prolonged antimicrobial therapy.
- ❖ Aggressive or advanced disease (facial nerve paralysis, bilateral involvement and advanced radiological findings such as bony destruction of the temporomandibular joint, soft tissue involvement in the infratemporal fossa or nasopharynx...).
- ❖ Facial nerve paralysis.
- ❖ Sterile deep-tissue culture.

Over time, the number of patients undergoing surgery has declined (50). This is due to the disappointing results of surgery, since it is often impossible to achieve complete exeresis of the lesions. On the other hand, surgery has been criticized for opening up new avenues of extension, promoting the spread of infection and increasing morbidity (141).

Currently, the role of surgery in OEN is adjuvant or complementary, and requires multidisciplinary consultation on a case-by-case basis. It consists of purely local procedures: removal of bone sequestration, debridement of infected tissues and drainage of purulent collections (59,61,142). Some authors do not recommend surgery for therapeutic purposes, but rather for etiological reasons in the event of biopsy and culture to differentiate ENT from neoplasia (31). Facial nerve decompression is no longer indicated for facial paralysis in patients with OEN (46).

Further data are needed to establish the role of surgery in the management of OEN (50).

CHAPTER 8:
MONITORING AND PREVENTION

1. MONITORING DURING TREATMENT

Regular patient monitoring is essential for early detection of complications. It is based on clinical, biological, bacteriological and radiological criteria (31,55,61,115).

1.1 Clinical monitoring

Daily monitoring. It consists of monitoring the intensity of otalgia, the abundance of otorrhea and the appearance of granulations on otoscopy.
A neurological examination is necessary to look for signs of localization, indicating endocranial extension.

1.2 Biological monitoring

It is based on monitoring changes in the kinetics of biological markers, notably C-reactive protein and sedimentation rate (21).
Glycemic control to ensure balanced diabetes is necessary for recovery (84,115).

1.3. Bacteriological monitoring

This monitoring is based on bacteriological samples taken regularly during the course of treatment until negativation is achieved.

1.4. Radiological monitoring

These criteria are essentially based on the normalization of gallium 67 scintigraphy. Most authors agree on the importance of the scintigraphic criterion, given that clinical and biological criteria are not always reliable (31,41). However, the high cost and difficulty of access to bone scintigraphy limit its use in the radiological assessment of OEN (96).
A recent article also mentions the value of the MRI diffusion sequence in patient follow-up: no irradiation and no injection of contrast medium in fragile patients with potential diabetic nephropathy. Indeed, the ADC (Apparent Diffusion Coefficient), abnormally high in inflammatory areas of the rock, normalizes during healing (143).

2. LONG-TERM MONITORING

Recurrence, up to a year after treatment, has been described in the literature in 15-20% of cases, so patients need to be monitored regularly during this period before they can be considered cured (20,46,52,144).

3. PREVENTION

Prevention is always the best treatment for OEN. Given that the majority of individuals developing OEN are diabetics who have suffered self-inflicted or iatrogenic trauma to the ear as a precipitating event, it is important to warn susceptible individuals about this. It is preferable not to manipulate the EAC even with cotton swabs (115,145). The diabetic patient must take care to optimize his or her lifestyle and diabetic balance, respecting treatments, dietary measures and the eradication of infectious sources, particularly dental and ENT (31). For people who are usually in the water, specific measures are needed to prevent OEN, including the use of earplugs, drying the ears by shaking them after swimming and using a hairdryer after exposure to water (setting the hairdryer at low speed and low temperature at least 30 cm from the ears) (145,146).

The physician also plays an important role in the prevention of OEN. Indeed, the otologist must observe certain precautions when handling the ear: auricular irrigation for earwax removal should be carried out with care by medical personnel, avoiding injury to the wall of the CAE (31). In the case of simple otitis externa, clinical and otoscopic monitoring after 48 to 72 hours of topical treatment is necessary to detect an unfavourable evolution and consequently suspect OEN (22,147).

CHAPTER 9: EVOLUTION

Thanks to better understanding of the disease and earlier diagnosis and appropriate treatment, the prognosis for ESO has improved in recent years, with increased survival rates (61,148).

1. HEALING

Patients are considered cured if they progress favorably after 12 months off treatment. An increased cure rate of up to 90% of patients has been reported in most series in the literature, thanks to new strategies adopted in the management of the disease (101,148-150).

2. COMPLICATIONS AND AFTER-EFFECTS

Complications of OEN arise from invasion of surrounding structures, principally the cranial nerves. Although the facial nerve is most frequently affected, other nerves may also be involved: the glossopharyngeal, vagus, spinal accessory, hypoglossal, trigeminal and abducens nerves. This damage may persist permanently, causing disabling aesthetic and functional sequelae (30,148):

- Facial paralysis is unsightly, interfering with phonation and eating, and can lead to corneal damage due to a lack of palpebral occlusion.
- Involvement of the mixed nerves can cause recurrent paralysis or pharyngeal constrictor paralysis, which may even be responsible for permanent total aphagia.

Osteomyelitis of the skull base occurs when the infection extends beyond the temporal bone and spreads to the sphenoid bone, occipital bone or clivus (88). Intracranial involvement can manifest as a range of symptoms from mild confusion to more serious conditions, including meningitis or venous sinus thrombosis (46).

3. RECIDIVE

According to published series, recurrence occurs in 10-20% of cases (53,150). Certain factors increase the risk of recurrence, such as advanced age, unbalanced diabetes, the presence of complications at diagnosis (facial paralysis, etc.) and short treatment duration (76). These recurrences can occur up to a year after antibiotics have been discontinued, necessitating regular and prolonged monitoring (46).

4. DEATH

Following the transition from aggressive surgery to antibiotic therapy based on fluoroquinolones and C3G, which have a broad spectrum and good intraosseous distribution, the mortality rate fell from 42% (13,144) to 15% (53,117). Some authors have even noted figures below 10% (20,24,151).

Mortality can be attributed to multiple factors, mainly: age over 70, systemic immunosuppression (including non-diabetic patients), intracranial complications or complications secondary to prolonged antibiotic treatment.

DECISION ALGORITHM

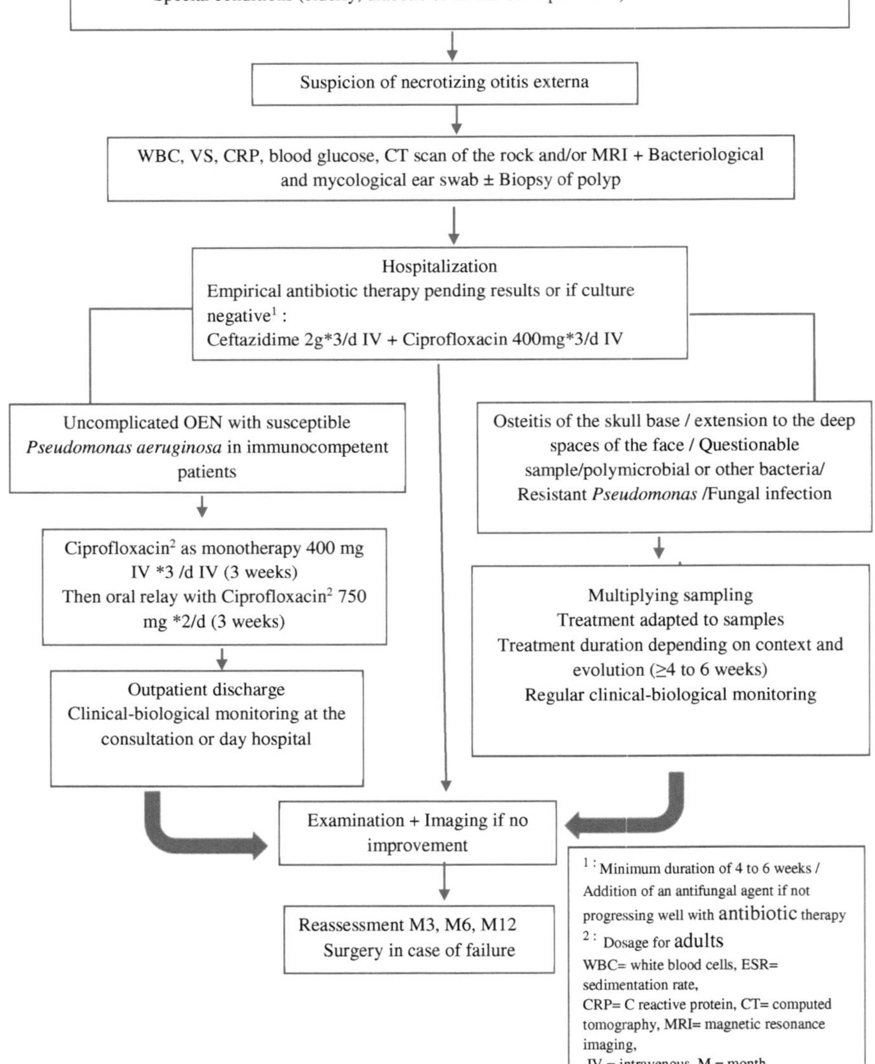

• Otitis externa resistant to local antibiotic treatment (≥7 days)
• Severe ear pain with a vesperal exacerbation resistant to minor analgesics and/or otorrhea refractory to ototopic treatments
• Granulation tissue in the floor of the external auditory canal on otoscopy
• Special conditions (elderly, diabetic or immunocompromised)
Suspicion of necrotizing otitis externa
WBC, VS, CRP, blood glucose, CT scan of the rock and/or MRI + Bacteriological and mycological ear swab ± Biopsy of polyp
Hospitalization
Empirical antibiotic therapy pending results or if culture negative[1] :
Ceftazidime 2g*3/d IV + Ciprofloxacin 400mg*3/d IV
Uncomplicated OEN with susceptible *Pseudomonas aeruginosa* in immunocompetent patients
Ciprofloxacin[2] as monotherapy 400 mg IV *3 /d IV (3 weeks)
Then oral relay with Ciprofloxacin[2] 750 mg *2/d (3 weeks)
Outpatient discharge
Clinical-biological monitoring at the consultation or day hospital
Osteitis of the skull base / extension to the deep spaces of the face / Questionable sample/polymicrobial or other bacteria/ Resistant *Pseudomonas* /Fungal infection
Multiplying sampling
Treatment adapted to samples
Treatment duration depending on context and evolution (≥4 to 6 weeks)
Regular clinical-biological monitoring
Examination + Imaging if no improvement
Reassessment M3, M6, M12
Surgery in case of failure
1 : Minimum duration of 4 to 6 weeks / Addition of an antifungal agent if not progressing well with antibiotic therapy
2 : Dosage for adults
WBC= white blood cells, ESR= sedimentation rate,
CRP= C reactive protein, CT= computed tomography, MRI= magnetic resonance imaging,
IV = intravenous, M = month

CONCLUSION

Necrotizing otitis externa is a serious infection of the external auditory canal, resulting in bone and cartilage necrosis that can spread to adjacent structures and be life-threatening.

Its pathogenesis is explained by the combination of a debilitating background: an elderly diabetic subject with diminished immune defenses, and an aggressive germ: *Pseudomonas aeruginosa* in the majority of cases. In recent years, however, we have noted a decrease in *Pseudomonas* cultures and a greater frequency of negative cultures.

An increase in the frequency of SDO in recent years has been noted in the literature, arousing growing interest in the medical community.

There is always a delay in diagnosis, as the lack of specificity of the clinical presentation makes it difficult to rapidly evoke OEN.

The initial work-up is based on a CT scan to detect bone lysis and/or an MRI scan to demonstrate osteitis and specify soft-tissue extension. Technetium 99-labelled diphosphonate bone scans, labelled leukocyte scans or, as recently proposed, PET CT scans may also be discussed.

Once the diagnosis has been confirmed, a multidisciplinary approach should be adopted, involving all the specialists concerned, in order to optimize the management of patients with OEN.

Optimization of diabetic control, and antibiotic therapy active against *Pseudomonas aeruginosa* with a combination of C3G and ciprofloxacin for an initial duration of 6 weeks would appear to be the most appropriate therapeutic approach. Hyperbaric oxygen therapy and surgery have no place in first-line treatment.

It's difficult to say whether a necrotizing otitis externa has been cured: the criteria for discontinuing antibiotic treatment are still not well established. They are essentially based on clinico-radiological data. Ga67 scintigraphy remains the reference examination in most centers. PET CT would be the ideal test for confirming treatment discontinuation, since it has 96% sensitivity and 91% specificity. Our study highlights the need for a future prospective and analytical study to better codify the therapeutic management of patients with OEN, by studying, in particular, the resistance profiles of the germs responsible for this condition, in order to highlight the recommended combinations of antibiotics and avoid therapeutic failures. A larger study would be more robust and would yield significant and useful results.

BIBLIOGRAPHY

1. Kaushik V, Malik T, Saeed SR. Interventions for acute otitis externa. Cochrane Database Syst Rev. 20 Jan 2010;(1):CD004740.
2. Meltzer PE, Kelemen G. Pyocyaneous osteomyelitis of the temporal bone, mandible and zygoma. The Laryngoscope. 1959;69(10):1300-16.
3. Lucente FE, Parisier SC. James R. Chandler: "Malignant external otitis." Laryngoscope. july 1996;106(7):805-7.
4. Ridder GJ, Breunig C, Kaminsky J, Pfeiffer J. Central skull base osteomyelitis: new insights and implications for diagnosis and treatment. Eur Arch Otorhinolaryngol. May 2015;272(5):1269-76.
5. Mahdyoun P, Pulcini C, Gahide I, Raffaelli C, Savoldelli C, Castillo L, et al. Necrotizing Otitis Externa: A Systematic Review. Otology & Neurotology. June 2013;34(4):620-9.
6. Loh, T. L., Renger, L., Latis, S., & Patel, H. Malignant otitis externa in Australian Aboriginal patients: A 9-year retrospective analysis from the Northern Territory. The Australian journal of rural health 2019. 27(1), 78-82.
7. Chen JC, Yeh CF, Shiao AS, Tu TY. Temporal Bone Osteomyelitis: The Relationship with Malignant Otitis Externa, the Diagnostic Dilemma, and Changing Trends. The Scientific World Journal. 2014;2014:1-10.
8. Hamzany Y, Soudry E, Preis M, Hadar T, Hilly O, Bishara J, et al. Fungal malignant external otitis. Journal of Infection. March 2011;62(3):226-31.
9. Chnitir. S. Necrotizing external otitis: about 45 cases. Thesis, Faculty of Medicine, Tunis. 2005.
10. Cheng Y, Yang T, Wu C, Kao Y, Shia B, Lin H. A population-based time trend study in the incidence of malignant otitis externa. Clinical Otolaryngology. sept 2019;44(5):851-5.

11.Guerrero-Espejo A, Valenciano-Moreno I, Ramírez-Llorens R, Pérez-Monteagudo P. Otitis externa maligna en España. Acta Otorrinolaringológica Española. jan 2017;68(1):23-8.

12. Arsovic N, Radivojevic N, Jesic S, Babac S, Cvorovic L, Dudvarski Z. Malignant Otitis Externa: Causes for Various Treatment Responses. J Int Adv Otol. Apr 2020;16(1):98-103.

13. Hatch JL, Bauschard MJ, Nguyen SA, Lambert PR, Meyer TA, McRackan TR. Malignant Otitis Externa Outcomes: A Study of the University HealthSystem Consortium Database. Ann Otol Rhinol Laryngol. August 2018;127(8):514-20.

14. Eweiss AZ, Al-Aaraj M, Sethukumar P, Jama G. Necrotizing otitis externa: a serious condition becoming more frequently encountered. J Laryngol Otol. May 2022;136(5):386-90.

15. Chawdhary G, Liow N, Democratis J, Whiteside O. Necrotising (malignant) otitis externa in the UK: a growing problem. Review of five cases and analysis of national Hospital Episode Statistics trends. J Laryngol Otol. June 2015;129(6):600-3.

16. Bhasker D, Hartley A, Agada F. Is Malignant Otitis Externa on the Increase? A Retrospective Review of Cases. Ear Nose Throat J. Feb 2017;96(2):E1-5.

17. Sylvester MJ, Sanghvi S, Patel VM, Eloy JA, Ying YM. Malignant otitis externa hospitalizations: Analysis of patient characteristics. The Laryngoscope. oct 2017;127(10):2328-36.

18. Treviño González JL, Reyes Suárez LL, Hernández De León JE. Malignant otitis externa: An updated review. American Journal of Otolaryngology. March 2021;42(2):102894.

19. Hutson KH, Watson GJ. Malignant otitis externa, an increasing burden in the twenty-first century: review of cases in a UK teaching hospital, with a proposed algorithm for diagnosis and management. J Laryngol Otol. May 2019;133(05):356-62.
20. Costa MB, Onishi ET. Necrotizing Otitis Externa: A Proposal for Diagnostic and Therapeutic Approach. Int Arch Otorhinolaryngol. Oct 2023;27(04):e706-12.
21. Abed.I. Les otites externes nécrosantes à propos de 43 cas.Thèse de médecine.Faculté de médecine de Sfax.2016.
22. Guevara N, Mahdyoun P, Pulcini C, Raffaelli C, Gahide I, Castillo L. Initial management of necrotizing external otitis: Errors to avoid. European Annals of Otorhinolaryngology, Head and Neck Diseases. June 2013;130(3):115-21.
23. Yigider AP, Ovunc O, Arslan E, Sunter AV, Cermik TF, Yigit O. Malignant Otitis Externa: How to Monitor the Disease in Outcome Estimation? Medeni Med J. 2021;36(1):23-29.
24. Sylvester MJ, Sanghvi S, Patel VM, Eloy JA, Ying YM. Malignant otitis externa hospitalizations: Analysis of patient characteristics. The Laryngoscope. oct 2017;127(10):2328-36.
25. Sideris G, Latzonis J, Avgeri C, Malamas V, Delides A, Nikolopoulos T. A Different Era for Malignant Otitis Externa: The Non-Diabetic and Non-Immunocompromised Patients. J Int Adv Otol. 2022 Jan;18(1):20-24
26. Yang TH, Xirasagar S, Cheng YF, Wu CS, Kao YW, Shia BC, et al. Malignant Otitis Externa is Associated with Diabetes: A Population-Based Case-Control Study. Ann Otol Rhinol Laryngol. June 2020;129(6):585-90.

27. Glikson E, Sagiv D, Wolf M, Shapira Y. Necrotizing otitis externa: diagnosis, treatment, and outcome in a case series. Diagnostic Microbiology and Infectious Disease. jan 2017;87(1):74-8.
28. Jennifer Rubin Grandis,Morven S Edwards, Marlene L Durand, Milana Bogorodskaya, Malignant (necrotizing) external otitis, UpToDate2024. Available July 4, 2024: Link: https://www.uptodate.com/contents/necrotizing-malignant-external-otitis
29. Guevara N, Mahdyoun P, Pulcini C, Raffaelli C, Gahide I, Castillo L. Initial management of necrotizing external otitis: Errors to avoid. European Annals of Otorhinolaryngology, Head and Neck Diseases. June 2013;130(3):115-21.
30. Bathokedeou A, Essobozou P, Akouda P, Essohanam B, Eyawelohn K. Epidemiological, clinical and therapeutical aspects of otitis externa: about 801 cases. Pan Afr Med J. 28 Feb 2014;17:142.
31 Kumar SP, Singh U. Malignant Otitis Externa-A Review. J Infect Dis Ther 3: 204 (2015).
32. Unadkat S, Kanzara T, Watters G. Necrotizing otitis externa in the immunocompetent patient: case series. J Laryngol Otol. Jan 2018;132(1):71-4.
33. Soudry E, Hamzany Y, Preis M, Joshua B, Hadar T, Nageris BI. Malignant External Otitis: Analysis of Severe Cases. Otolaryngol-head neck surg. May 2011;144(5):758-62.
34 Long DA, Koyfman A, Long B. An emergency medicine-focused review of malignant otitis externa. The American Journal of Emergency Medicine. August 2020;38(8):1671-8.
35 Mani N, Sudhoff H, Rajagopal S, Moffat D, Axon PR. Cranial Nerve Involvement in Malignant External Otitis: Implications for Clinical Outcome. The Laryngoscope. May 2007;117(5):907-10.

36. Berenholz L, Katzenell U, Harell M. Evolving Resistant Pseudomonas to Ciprofloxacin in Malignant Otitis Externa. The Laryngoscope. Sept 2002;112(9):1619-22.
37. 10.1007/s12070-018-1426-0 TA, Adeagbo AK. The Association Between Malignant Otitis Externa and Diabetes Mellitus in Africa: A Systematic Review. Indian J Otolaryngol Head Neck Surg. Dec 2023;75(4):3277-87.
38. Peled C, Sadeh R, El-Saied S, Novack V, Kaplan DM. Diabetes and glycemic control in necrotizing otitis externa (NOE). Eur Arch Otorhinolaryngol. March 2022;279(3):1269-75.
39. C, El-Seid S, Bahat-Dinur A, Tzvi-Ran LR, Kraus M, Kaplan D. Necrotizing Otitis Externa-Analysis of 83 Cases: Clinical Findings and Course of Disease. Otology & Neurotology. jan 2019;40(1):56-62.
40. Byun YJ, Patel J, Nguyen SA, Lambert PR. Necrotizing Otitis Externa: A Systematic Review and Analysis of Changing Trends. Otology & Neurotology. Sept 2020;41(8):1004-11.
41. Hu L, Gao X, Wang X, Xu J, Wang X. [Research progress of necrotizing otitis externa]. Lin Chuang Er Bi Yan Hou Tou Jing Wai Ke Za Zhi. 2023 Oct;37(10):843-847;852. Chinese.
42 Joshua BZ, Sulkes J, Raveh E, Bishara J, Nageris BI. Predicting Outcome of Malignant External Otitis. Otology & Neurotology. Apr 2008;29(3):339-43.
43. Stern Shavit S, Soudry E, Hamzany Y, Nageris B. Malignant external otitis: Factors predicting patient outcomes. American Journal of Otolaryngology. sept 2016;37(5):425-30.
44. Lee SK, Lee SA, Seon SW, Jung JH, Lee JD, Choi JY, et al. Analysis of Prognostic Factors in Malignant External Otitis. Clin Exp Otorhinolaryngol. 1 Sep 2017;10(3):228-35.

45. Loh S, Loh WS. Malignant otitis externa: an Asian perspective on treatment outcomes and prognostic factors. Otolaryngol Head Neck Surg. 2013 Jun;148(6):991-6
46. Al Aaraj MS, Kelley C. Necrotizing (Malignant) Otitis Externa. [Updated 2023 Oct 29]. In: StatPearls. Treasure Island (FL): StatPearls Publishing; 2024 Jan. https://www.ncbi.nlm.nih.gov/books/NBK556138/
47. Walton J, Coulson C. Fungal malignant otitis externa with facial nerve palsy: tissue biopsy AIDS diagnosis. Case Rep Otolaryngol. 2014;2014:192318.
48. Orioli L, Boute C, Eloy P, De Wispelaere JF, De Coene B, Huang TD, et al. Central skull base osteomyelitis: a rare but life-threatening disease. Acta Clinica Belgica. August 1, 2015;70(4):291-4.
49. Liu XL, Peng H, Mo TT, Liang Y. Malignant otitis externa in a healthy non-diabetic patient. Eur Arch Otorhinolaryngol. August 2016;273(8):2261-5.
50. Takata J, Hopkins M, Alexander V, Bannister O, Dalton L, Harrison L, et al. Systematic review of the diagnosis and management of necrotizing otitis externa: Highlighting the need for high-quality research. Clinical Otolaryngology. 2023;48(3):381-94.
51. Bruschini L, Berrettini S, Christina C, Ferranti S, Fabiani S, Cavezza M, Forli F, Santoro A, Tagliaferri E. Extensive Skull Base Osteomyelitis Secondary to Malignant Otitis Externa. J Int Adv Otol. 2019 Dec;15(3):463-465.
52. Lau K, Scotta G, Wu K, Kabuli MAK, Watson G. A review of thirty-nine patients diagnosed with necrotizing otitis externa over three years: Is CT imaging for diagnosis sufficient? Clinical Otolaryngology. May 2020;45(3):414-8.

53. Mahdyoun P, Pulcini C, Gahide I, Raffaelli C, Savoldelli C, Castillo L, et al. Necrotizing Otitis Externa: A Systematic Review. Otology & Neurotology. June 2013;34(4):620-9.
54. Marina S, Goutham MK, Rajeshwary A, Vadisha B, Devika T. A retrospective review of 14 cases of malignant otitis externa. Journal of Otology. June 2019;14(2):63-6.
55. Honnurappa V, Ramdass S, Mahajan N, Vijayendra VK, Redleaf M. Effective Inexpensive Management of Necrotizing Otitis Externa Is Possible in Resource-Poor Settings. Ann Otol Rhinol Laryngol. Sept 2019;128(9):848-54.
56. Hasibi M, Ashtiani MK, Motassadi Zarandi M, Yazdani N, Borghei P, Kuhi A, et al. A Treatment Protocol for Management of Bacterial and Fungal Malignant External Otitis: A Large Cohort in Tehran, Iran. Ann Otol Rhinol Laryngol. 1 Jul 2017;126(7):561-7.
57. Sekar R, Raja K, Ganesan S, Alexander A, Saxena SK. Clinical and Current Microbiological Profile with Changing Antibiotic Sensitivity in Malignant Otitis Externa. Indian J Otolaryngol Head Neck Surg. Dec 2022;74(Suppl 3):4422-7.
58. Byun YJ, Patel J, Nguyen SA, Lambert PR. Hyperbaric oxygen therapy in malignant otitis externa: A systematic review of the literature. World j otorhinolaryngol-head neck surg. oct 2021;7(4):296-302.
59. Lambor DV, Das CP, Goel HC, Tiwari M, Lambor SD, Fegade MV. Necrotizing otitis externa: clinical profile and management protocol. J Laryngol Otol. nov 2013;127(11):1071-7.
60. Singh J, Bhardwaj B. The Role of Surgical Debridement in Cases of Refractory Malignant Otitis Externa. Indian J Otolaryngol Head Neck Surg. 2018;70(4):549-54.

61. Mahdyoun P, Pulcini C, Gahide I, Raffaelli C, Savoldelli C, Castillo L, et al. Necrotizing Otitis Externa: A Systematic Review. Otology & Neurotology. June 2013;34(4):620-9.

62. Balakrishnan R, Dalakoti P, Nayak DR, Pujary K, Singh R, Kumar R. Efficacy of HRCT Imaging vs SPECT/CT Scans in the Staging of Malignant External Otitis. Otolaryngol--head neck surg. August 2019;161(2):336-42.

63. Migirov L, Lipshitz N, Dagan E, Wolf M. Is laterality of malignant otitis externa related to handedness? Med Hypotheses. Jul 2013;81(1):142-3.

64. H. Moata, G. EL Mghari , N.EL Ansari, R.Ait el abdia, Y.Rochdi, H.Nouri, L.Aderdour and A.Raji. Les otites necrosantes: lorsque l'hyperglycemie prend sa part: a propos de 32 cas. Int. J. of Adv. Res 2019; 7 (Jan). 394-399.

65. Khan MA, Quadri SAQ, Kazmi AS, Kwatra V, Ramachandran A, Gustin A, et al. A Comprehensive Review of Skull Base Osteomyelitis: Diagnostic and Therapeutic Challenges among Various Presentations. Asian J Neurosurg. 2018;13(4):959-70.

66 Stevens SM, Lambert PR, Baker AB, Meyer TA. Malignant Otitis Externa: A Novel Stratification Protocol for Predicting Treatment Outcomes. Otol Neurotol. Sept 2015;36(9):1492-8.

67. Kamalden TMIT, Misron K. A 10-year review of malignant otitis externa: a new insight. Eur Arch Otorhinolaryngol. June 2022;279(6):2837-44.

68. van Kroonenburgh AMJL, van der Meer WL, Bothof RJP, van Tilburg M, van Tongeren J, Postma AA. Advanced Imaging Techniques in Skull Base Osteomyelitis Due to Malignant Otitis Externa. Curr Radiol Rep. 2018;6(1):3.

69. Karaman E, Yilmaz M, Ibrahimov M, Haciyev Y, Enver O. Malignant otitis externa. J Craniofac Surg. nov 2012;23(6):1748-51.

70. Zonnour A, Jamshidi A, Dabiri S, Hasibi M, Tajdini A, Karrabi N, et al. Predictive factors in treatment response of malignant external otitis. Eur Arch Otorhinolaryngol. 1 Jan 2023;280(1):159-66.
71. Peled C, Kraus M, Kaplan D. Diagnosis and treatment of necrotizing otitis externa and diabetic foot osteomyelitis - similarities and differences. J Laryngol Otol. Sept 2018;132(9):775-9.
72. McLaren O, Potter C. Scedosporium apiospermum: a rare cause of malignant otitis externa. BMJ Case Rep. 9 Sep 2016;2016:bcr2016217015.
73. Gruber M, Roitman A, Doweck I, Uri N, Shaked-Mishan P, Kolop-Feldman A, et al. Clinical Utility of a Polymerase Chain Reaction Assay in Culture-Negative Necrotizing Otitis Externa. Otology & Neurotology. Apr 2015;36(4):733-6.
74. Kozel TR, Wickes B. Fungal diagnostics. Cold Spring Harb Perspect Med. 1 Apr 2014;4(4):a019299.
75. Hobson CE, Moy JD, Byers KE, Raz Y, Hirsch BE, McCall AA. Malignant Otitis Externa: Evolving Pathogens and Implications for Diagnosis and Treatment. Otolaryngology-Head and Neck Surgery. 2014;151(1):112-6.
76. Chabbert.S.Otite externe nécrosante:évaluation globale d'une prise en charge dans un center hospitalouniversitaire avec analyse des échecs thérapeutiques. Thèse d'exercixe en médecine . Université Claude Bernard Lyon 1.2017
77. Marchionni E, Parize P, Lefevre A, Vironneau P, Bougnoux ME, Poiree S, et al. Aspergillus spp. invasive external otitis: favorable outcome with a medical approach. Clinical Microbiology and Infection. May 2016;22(5):434-7.

78. Marchionni E, Parize P, Lefevre A, Vironneau P, Bougnoux ME, Poiree S, et al. Aspergillus spp. invasive external otitis: favorable outcome with a medical approach. Clinical Microbiology and Infection. May 2016;22(5):434-7.
79. Halwani C, Mtibaa L, Hamdi ME, Baccouchi N, Benmhamed R, Jemli B, Akkari K. A retrospective study of 43 cases of fungal malignant external otitis. Pan Afr Med J. 2022 Apr 8;41:287.
80. QASIM ZS, . Sensitivity of Fungi Isolated from Patients Infected with Otitis Externa by Using Antifungal Drugs. J.Res.Pharm. 2023; 27(6): 2548-2558.
81. Lotfali E , Ghasemi R, Masoumi N, Molavizadeh D, Sadeghi S, et al. Isolation, Characterization, and Antifungal Sensitivity Pattern of Fungal Species with Potential Resistance to Antifungal Drugs in Patients with Otomycosis. Arch Clin Infect Dis. 2022;17(4):e129169.
82. Kiakojuri K, Mahdavi Omran S, Roodgari S, Taghizadeh Armaki M, Hedayati MT, Shokohi T, et al. Molecular Identification and Antifungal Susceptibility of Yeasts and Molds Isolated from Patients with Otomycosis. Mycopathologia. May 2021;186(2):245-57.
83. Peled C, Parra A, El-saied S, Kraus M, Kaplan DM. Surgery for necrotizing otitis externa-indications and surgical findings. Eur Arch Otorhinolaryngol. May 2020;277(5):1327-34.
84. Hopkins ME, Bennett A, Henderson N, MacSween KF, Baring D, Sutherland R. A retrospective review and multi-specialty, evidence-based guideline for the management of necrotizing otitis externa. J Laryngol Otol. June 2020;134(6):487-92.
85. Peled C, Kraus M, Kaplan D. Diagnosis and treatment of necrotizing otitis externa and diabetic foot osteomyelitis - similarities and differences. J Laryngol Otol. Sept 2018;132(9):775-9.

86. Stern Shavit S, Bernstine H, Sopov V, Nageris B, Hilly O. FDG-PET/CT for diagnosis and follow-up of necrotizing (malignant) external otitis. Laryngoscope. 2019 Apr;129(4):961-966.
87. Salaheddine H. Malignant otitis externa about 20 cases. Thesis from the Faculty of Medicine and Pharmacy Marrakech. 2015.
88. Van Kroonenburgh AMJL, Van Der Meer WL, Bothof RJP, Van Tilburg M, Van Tongeren J, Postma AA. Advanced Imaging Techniques in Skull Base Osteomyelitis Due to Malignant Otitis Externa. Curr Radiol Rep. Jan 2018;6(1):3.
89. Van Der Meer WL, Waterval JJ, Kunst HPM, Mitea C, Pegge SAH, Postma AA. Diagnosing necrotizing external otitis on CT and MRI: assessment of pattern of extension. Eur Arch Otorhinolaryngol. March 2022;279(3):1323-8.
90. Cooper T, Hildrew D, McAfee JS, McCall AA, Branstetter BF, Hirsch BE. Imaging in the Diagnosis and Management of Necrotizing Otitis Externa: A Survey of Practice Patterns. Otol Neurotol. June 2018;39(5):597-601.
91. Balakrishnan R, Dalakoti P, Nayak DR, Pujary K, Singh R, Kumar R. Efficacy of HRCT Imaging vs SPECT/CT Scans in the Staging of Malignant External Otitis. Otolaryngol--head neck surg. August 2019;161(2):336-42.
92. Lau K, Scotta G, Wu K, Kabuli MAK, Watson G. A review of thirty-nine patients diagnosed with necrotizing otitis externa over three years: Is CT imaging for diagnosis sufficient? Clinical Otolaryngology. May 2020;45(3):414-8.
93. Khan HA. Necrotizing Otitis Externa: A Review of Imaging Modalities. Cureus. 2021. 13(12):e20675.

94. Kim DH, Kim SW, Hwang SH. Predictive value of radiologic studies for malignant otitis externa: a systematic review and meta-analysis. Brazilian Journal of Otorhinolaryngology. Jan 2023;89(1):66-72.
95. Galletti F, Cammaroto G, Galletti B, Quartuccio N, Di Mauro F, Baldari S. Technetium-99m (^{99} mTc)-labelled sulesomab in the management of malignant external otitis: is there any role? Eur Arch Otorhinolaryngol. June 2015;272(6):1377-82.
96. Sturm JJ, Stern Shavit S, Lalwani AK. What is the Best Test for Diagnosis and Monitoring Treatment Response in Malignant Otitis Externa? The Laryngoscope. Nov 2020;130(11):2516-7.
97. Goh JPN, Karandikar A, Loke SC, Tan TY. Skull base osteomyelitis secondary to malignant otitis externa mimicking advanced nasopharyngeal cancer: MR imaging features at initial presentation. Am J Otolaryngol. 2017;38(4):466-71.
98. Cohen D, Friedman P. The diagnostic criteria of malignant external otitis. J Laryngol Otol. March 1987;101(3):216-21.
99. Corey JP, Levandowski RA, Panwalker AP. Prognostic implications of therapy for necrotizing external otitis. Am J Otol. July 1985;6(4):353-8.
100. Levenson MJ, Parisier SC, Dolitsky J, Bindra G. Ciprofloxacin: drug of choice in the treatment of malignant external otitis (MEO). Laryngoscope. August 1991;101(8):821-4.
101. Bruno G, Valentina KM, Santoro R, Cammaroto G, Galletti F, Cascio A. Malignant external otitis. A case series from an Italian Tertiary-Care Hospital. Acta Med Mediter. 2014;30(6):1317-23.
102. Thakar A, Tandon DA, Bahadur S, Kacker SK. Malignant external otitis. IJO & HNS. Apr 1, 1996;48(2):114-20.

103. Kaya İ, Sezgin B, Eraslan S, Öztürk K, Göde S, Bilgen C, et al. Malignant Otitis Externa: A Retrospective Analysis and Treatment Outcomes. Turk Arch Otorhinolaryngol. June 2018;56(2):106-10.

104 Pritchett CV, Thorne MC. Incidence of pediatric acute mastoiditis: 1997-2006. Arch Otolaryngol Head Neck Surg. May 2012;138(5):451-5.

105. Majeed J, Sudarshan Reddy L. Role of CT Mastoids in the Diagnosis and Surgical Management of Chronic Inflammatory Ear Diseases. Indian J Otolaryngol Head Neck Surg. march 2017;69(1):113-20.

106. Barkanova ON, Николаевна БО, Gagarina SG, Г ГС, Kaluzhenina AA, A КА. Tuberculous medium otitis: clinical example. Journal of Volgograd State Medical University. 15 Apr 2020;17(4):103-5.

107. Hand, J. M., & Pankey, G. A. Tuberculous Otomastoiditis. Microbiology spectrum, 4(6), 10.1128/microbiolspec.TNMI7-0020-2016.

108. Hertz J, Siim C. External auditory canal cholesteatoma and benign necrotizing otitis externa: clinical study of 95 cases in the Capital Region of Denmark. J Laryngol Otol. June 2018;132(06):514-8.

109. Loock J. Keratosis obturans and external ear cholesteatoma. Clinical Otolaryngology. Apr 2005;30(2):213-213.

110. Spilsbury K, Miller I, Semmens JB, Lannigan FJ. Factors associated with developing cholesteatoma: A study of 45,980 children with middle ear disease. The Laryngoscope. March 2010;120(3):625-30.

111. Trimarchi M, Sinico RA, Teggi R, Bussi M, Specks U, Meroni PL. Otorhinolaryngological manifestations in granulomatosis with polyangiitis (Wegener's). Autoimmunity Reviews. feb 2013;12(4):501-5.

112. Wojciechowska J, Krajewski W, Krajewski P, Kręcicki T. Granulomatosis With Polyangiitis in Otolaryngologist Practice: A Review of Current Knowledge. Clin Exp Otorhinolaryngol. March 7, 2016;9(1):8-13.

113. Thiagarajah R, Chapman P, Irvine A. Malignant otitis externa or malignancy: Report of two cases. European Journal of Radiology Extra. 1 Jul 2008;67(1):9-12.
114. Rainsbury P, Mitchell-Innes A, Wilson H, Prior M. Aspergilloma of the middle ear mimicking necrotizing otitis externa: case report. J Laryngol Otol. Nov 2010;124(11):1209-11.
115. Tsilivigkos C, Avramidis K, Ferekidis E, Doupis J. Malignant External Otitis: What the Diabetes Specialist Should Know-A Narrative Review. Diabetes Ther. Apr 2023;14(4):629-38.
116. Saravanam P, Ravikumar A, Somu L, Ismail N. Malignant otitis externa: An emerging scourge. Journal of Clinical Gerontology and Geriatrics. 1 Dec 2013;4:128-31.
117. Carlton DA, Perez EE, Smouha EE. Malignant external otitis: The shifting treatment paradigm. Am J Otolaryngol. 2018;39(1):41-5.
118. Karaiskos I, Lagou S, Pontikis K, Rapti V, Poulakou G. The "Old" and the "New" Antibiotics for MDR Gram-Negative Pathogens: For Whom, When, and How. Front Public Health. 2019;7:151.
119. Fang CH, Sun J, Jyung RW. Malignant otitis externa. Ear Nose Throat J. 2015;94(4-5):136-8.
120. Hariga I, Mardassi A, Belhaj Younes F, Ben Amor M, Zribi S, Ben Gamra O, et al. Necrotizing otitis externa: 19 cases' report. Eur Arch Otorhinolaryngol. August 2010;267(8):1193-8.
121. Pulcini C, Mahdyoun P, Cua E, Gahide I, Castillo L, Guevara N. Antibiotic therapy in necrotizing external otitis: case series of 32 patients and review of the literature. Eur J Clin Microbiol Infect Dis. Dec 2012;31(12):3287-94.

122. Bodilsen J, Brouwer MC, Nielsen H, Van De Beek D. Anti-infective treatment of brain abscess. Expert Rev Anti Infect Ther. Jul 2018;16(7):565-78.
123. Tunkel AR, Hasbun R, Bhimraj A, Byers K, Kaplan SL, Scheld WM, et al. 2017 Infectious Diseases Society of America's Clinical Practice Guidelines for Healthcare-Associated Ventriculitis and Meningitis. Clin Infect Dis. March 15, 2017;64(6):e34-65.
124. Courson AM, Vikram HR, Barrs DM. What are the criteria for terminating treatment for necrotizing (malignant) otitis externa: Necrotizing Otitis Externa: Ending Treatment. The Laryngoscope. Feb 2014;124(2):361-2.
125. Ciorba A, Cultrera R, Di Laora A, Grilli A, Bianchini C, Aimoni C. Malignant otitis externa in the antibiotic resistance era: key to successful treatment. B-ENT. 2018. 14:119-123
126. Peled C, El-Seid S, Bahat-Dinur A, Tzvi-Ran LR, Kraus M, Kaplan D. Necrotizing Otitis Externa-Analysis of 83 Cases: Clinical Findings and Course of Disease. Otology & Neurotology. jan 2019;40(1):56-62.
127. Parize P, Chandesris MO, Lanternier F, Poirée S, Viard JP, Bienvenu B, et al. Antifungal Therapy of Aspergillus Invasive Otitis Externa: Efficacy of Voriconazole and Review. Antimicrob Agents Chemother. March 2009;53(3):1048-53.
128. Pichon M, Joly V, Argy N, Houze S, Bretagne S, Alanio A, et al. Aspergillus flavus malignant external otitis in a diabetic patient: case report and literature review. Infection. Apr 2020;48(2):193-203.
129. Mion M, Bovo R, Marchese-Ragona R, Martini A. Outcome predictors of treatment effectiveness for fungal malignant external otitis: a systematic review. Acta Otorhinolaryngol Ital. oct 2015;35(5):307-13.

130. Maertens JA, Raad II, Marr KA, Patterson TF, Kontoyiannis DP, Cornely OA, et al. Isavuconazole versus voriconazole for primary treatment of invasive mould disease caused by Aspergillus and other filamentous fungi: a phase 3, randomised-controlled, non-inferiority trial. Lancet. Feb 20, 2016;387(10020):760-9.

131. Patterson TF, Thompson GR, Denning DW, Fishman JA, Hadley S, Herbrecht R, et al. Practice Guidelines for the Diagnosis and Management of Aspergillosis: 2016 Update by the Infectious Diseases Society of America. Clinical Infectious Diseases. August 15, 2016;63(4):e1-60.

132. Carfrae MJ, Kesser BW. Malignant otitis externa. Otolaryngol Clin North Am. June 2008;41(3):537-49, viii-ix.

133. Kaushik V, Malik T, Saeed SR. Interventions for acute otitis externa. Cochrane Database Syst Rev. 2010 Jan 20;(1):CD004740.

134. Llor C, McNulty CAM, Butler CC. Ordering and interpreting ear swabs in otitis externa. BMJ. Sep 1, 2014;349(sep01 2):g5259-g5259.

135. Bock K, Ovesen T. Optimised diagnosis and treatment of necrotizing external otitis is warranted. Dan Med Bull. Jul 2011;58(7):A4292.

136 Phillips JS, Jones SE. Hyperbaric oxygen as an adjuvant treatment for malignant otitis externa. Cochrane Database Syst Rev. 2013 May 31;2013(5):CD004617.

137. Savvidou OD, Kaspiris A, Bolia IK, Chloros GD, Goumenos SD, Papagelopoulos PJ, et al. Effectiveness of Hyperbaric Oxygen Therapy for the Management of Chronic Osteomyelitis: A Systematic Review of the Literature. Orthopedics. 1 Jul 2018;41(4):193-9.

138. Belchadi, M & Khereddine, N & Mani, Ramya & Chahed, H & Zeglaoui, I & ben ali, Meryem & Abdelkefi, M & Shiri, N & Bouzouita, K. L'Otite externe necorsante: Place de l'oxygenotherapie hyperbare.J. Tun ORL - N° 20.21-24. Juin2008.

139. Al Siyabi A, Al Farsi B, Al-Shidhani A, Al Hinai Z, Al Balushi Y, Al Qartoobi H. Management of Malignant Otitis Externa with Hyperbaric Oxygen Therapy: A Case Series of 20 Patients. Oman Med J. May 31, 2023;38(3):e512-e512.
140. Peled C, Parra A, El-saied S, Kraus M, Kaplan DM. Surgery for necrotizing otitis externa-indications and surgical findings. Eur Arch Otorhinolaryngol. May 2020;277(5):1327-34.
141. Galletti B, Mannella valentina katia, Santoro R, Cammaroto G, Freni F, Galletti F, et al. Malignant external otitis. A case series from an Italian Tertiary-Care Hospital. Acta Medica Mediterranea. 19 June 2014;2014:1317.
142. Kuczkowski J, Nowicki TK. Indications for surgery in necrotizing otitis externa. Eur Arch Otorhinolaryngol. June 2022;279(6):3219-20.
143. Cherko M, Nash R, Singh A, Lingam RK. Diffusion-weighted Magnetic Resonance Imaging as a Novel Imaging Modality in Assessing Treatment Response in Necrotizing Otitis Externa. Otol Neurotol. Jul 2016;37(6):704-7.
144. Amaro CE, Espiney R, Radu L, Guerreiro F. Malignant (necrotizing) externa otitis: the experience of a single hyperbaric center. Eur Arch Otorhinolaryngol. Jul 2019;276(7):1881-7.
145. Laura A Goguen, Marlene L Durand, Daniel G Deschler, FACS, Morven S Edwards, Jane Givens. External otitis: Treatment, UpToDate2023. Available June 12, 2024: https://www.uptodate.com/contents/external-otitis-in-adults-treatment
146. Wingelaar TT, van Ooij PJA, van Hulst RA. Otitis externa in military divers: more frequent and less harmful than reported. Diving Hyperb Med. March 2017;47(1):4-8.

147. Rosenfeld, R. M., Schwartz, S. R., Cannon, C. R., Roland, P. S., Simon, G. R., Kumar, K. A., Huang, W. W., Haskell, H. W., & Robertson, P. J. (2014). Clinical practice guideline: acute otitis externa. Otolaryngology--head and neck surgery: official journal of American Academy of Otolaryngology-Head and Neck Surgery, 150(1 Suppl), S1-S24.

148 Johnson AK, Batra PS. Central skull base osteomyelitis: An emerging clinical entity. The Laryngoscope. May 2014;124(5):1083-7.

149. Ahmed M, Syed R, More YI, Basha SI. Stenotrophomonas skull base osteomyelitis presenting as necrotizing otitis externa: Unmasking by CT and MRI-case report and review. Radiol Case Rep 2019 Oct; 14(10): 1241-1245.

150. Hasnaoui M, Ben Mabrouk A, Chelli J, Larbi Ammari F, Lahmar R, Toumi A, et al. Necrotising otitis externa: A single center experience. J Otol. Jan 2021;16(1):22-6.

151.Al-Noury K, Lotfy A. Computed tomography and magnetic resonance imaging findings before and after treatment of patients with malignant external otitis. Eur Arch Otorhinolaryngol. Dec 2011;268(12):1727-3

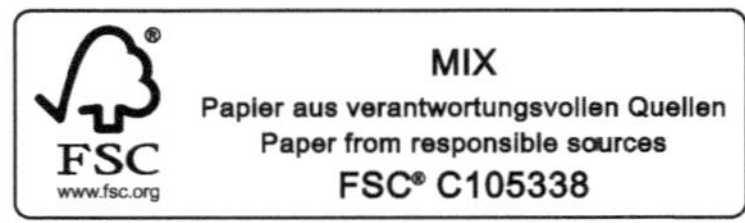

Printed by Books on Demand GmbH, Norderstedt / Germany